The Drir   ⧽

Everything your mother   *eeding*

Veronika Sophia Robinson

The Drinks Are On Me
Everything your mother never told you about breastfeeding
Veronika Sophia Robinson

© 2007

Published by
The Art of Change,
PO Box 441, East Grinstead, West Sussex
RH18 5DH
United Kingdom
www.artofchange.co.uk

ISBN:
0-9530063-4-4
978-0-9530063-4-2

Cover photographs by Marshall Lefferts
Pakiri beach pregnancy, breastfeeding and wedding photographs by Marshall Lefferts.

Other photography courtesy of Cindy Beaudin pp 60 & 88; Elizabeth Coldwell-Hall pp 27 & 106; and David Hollins, pp 147 and back cover gardening photo.

Illustrations by Andri Thwaites - except Nips, by Eliza Robinson, page 73; Udder One, by Stephen Carney, page 101; and Love Nest, by Maya Hayward, page 126.

Also by the same author
Fields of Lavender ~ collection of poetry
The Compassionate Years ~ a history of the RSPCA in New Zealand
Howl at the Moon (contributing poet)

Author's intention
The information contained in this book does not constitute medical advice. It is presented in good faith as a source of information to inspire and educate other families to make informed decisions; to take responsibility for their own, and their family's, health and well-being. The author can in no way be held liable for the choices readers make.

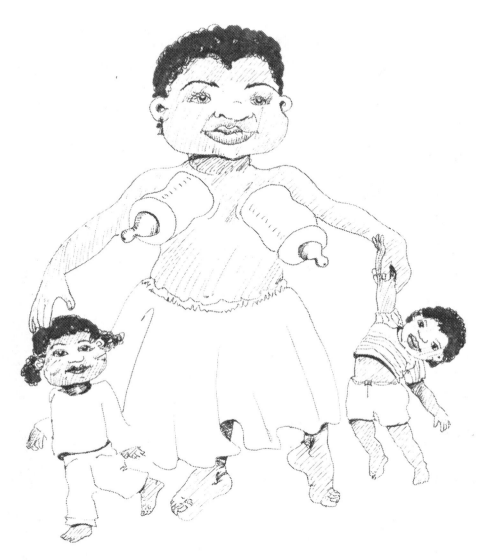

Dedication

This book is dedicated to the memory of the 4,000 babies who die *every day* because of artificial milk fed to them in bottles ~ and their mothers, who live out their lives with empty, aching hearts and empty arms. This global tragedy shows us the insanity of ignoring nature.

Contents

Happy Hour

My dad, **Albert Harbers**, for providing my childhood with a haven of mammals! You gifted me with so much, but it's only now, mid-life, that I can truly see how blessed I was.

Andri Thwaites, for capturing my thoughts into illustrations. Thank you.

Angelikah Om' Namaha, my beautiful mother, the woman who introduced me to breastfeeding. How could I have possibly chosen anyone else to be my mother? The gift you gave us while Eliza was in NICU is beyond words. No matter how many oceans separate us, you're always just a heart beat away.

Barbara Sheppard and **Paula Lernelius** at the former Lakeland La Leche League. Thank you for all your support.

Barbara Sturmfels at Central Auckland LLL, for opening my eyes and heart to full-term breastfeeding.

Barry & Winnie Durdant-Hollamby at The Art of Change publishing house, for believing in this book, and offering to publish, based on the title alone! You're my personal Fairy Godparents. And thank you to their daughters, **Anna** and **Sophie**, for sharing their parents and their unusual strategies, with me and my passions.

Bethany Angelika Robinson, for declaring to a disbelieving UK public that *"breast milk is better than a million melons, better than mango, even."* I'll always treasure those magical breastfeeding moments with you, my first born.

Cindy Beaudin, for standing out like a beacon at a La Leche League meeting and joining my journey in life as a true kindred spirit; and for publishing The Mother magazine in New Zealand. When I think of friendship, I think of you.

Eliza Serena Robinson, your first words to me were "I love you". Actually, it was more like "I uv ooooo"....but you clearly learnt it at my breast after a long night of croup.

Emma Lewis, a kindred spirit and passionate advocate for listening to the needs of the child. Thank you so much for reading the raw manuscript of this book and being supportive.

Gaylene Wickham, for encouraging me to go to La Leche League meetings. You were right, I did find like-minded people, and it changed my life.

The late, GREAT **Jeannine Parvati Baker,** America's favourite midwife, author, visionary and sacred birth-keeper, for all the conversations we shared, which brought insights and clarity to me, personally and professionally. Your wisdom will remain with us forever in the early editions of The Mother magazine. You are the brightest star in the sky, and I miss you deeply. Your untimely passing still brings tears to my eyes, and a lump to my throat. You left this world a better place!

Katie Buchanan, for bringing the message of full-term breastfeeding out into the public and pushing me well and truly out of my comfort zone. I still haven't worked out if I should be thanking you for it! I think you're gorgeous though.

Lynda Cook Sawyer, lactation consultant, fab friend and personal jester. MYNBTOTS!

Madhu Bhana, a wonderful cranio-sacral therapist on Auckland's North Shore, New Zealand. You are, to my family, an angel. We will never forget your care and kindness, not just in helping Eliza enormously in NICU, but for the months that followed in 'keeping us going', as you called it. We love you.

Marshall Lefferts, thank you so much for photographing my family, and capturing our breastfeeding and pregnancy memories for us.

My soul-mate, **Paul Robinson,** a bosom buddy to Bethany and Eliza. Thanks for finding a title for this book which fits perfectly. Thank you for lighting up every corner of my life with your humour, love, compassion and wisdom. Thank you for supporting me in my 'truth'. And, as ever, being a proof-reader to every piece of writing which leaves my finger tips. You, my love, have made my life.

Ruth Davison, midwife for Bethany's birth, for allowing us to birth and breastfeed naturally, and supporting our vision in setting up the NZ National Waterbirth Trust.

Sian Burgess, midwife for Eliza's birth, for introducing me to the term Liquid Love when describing breast milk, and for lighting up my family's life with the story of *Bash me with the Boobas.* It's brought so much laughter.

Tish Clifford, for understanding the vital importance of DHA to the human brain, and being a sounding board to my passion.

The numerous mothers whose wisdom, insights and knowledge opened my eyes to worlds unseen, inspiring me to follow my heart and my daughters' cues. Thank you for having the courage to speak out.

To every breastfeeding mum I've had the pleasure of witnessing feed her baby naturally. Each time, a song danced through my heart, and I went "YES!"

No author can ever claim to write a book on their own. So many people pass through our life, heart and thoughts as they imprint a bit of themselves onto us. We take these threads and weave them into our being, then spread a blanket out into the world in the hope it might provide warmth and comfort to others. For the many, many people who've shared moments of time in my life, and contributed to me opening up to more of myself, I thank you.

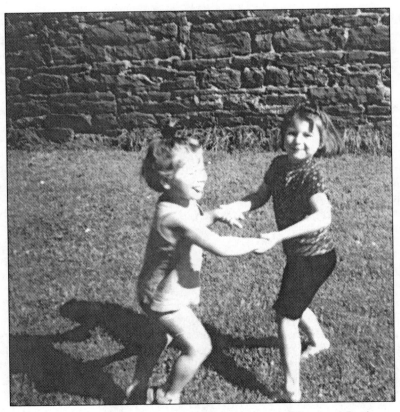

My beautiful, gorgeous, love-filled shadows, Eliza and Bethany. Cumbria 2000

Shadows

Author unknown

I saw a young mother
With eyes full of laughter
And two little shadows
Came following after

Wherever she moved
They were always right there
Holding onto her skirts
Hanging onto her chair
Before her, behind her
An adhesive pair

"Don't you ever get weary
As day after day
Your two little tagalongs
Get in your way?"

She smiled as she shook
Her pretty young head
And I'll always remember
the words that she said:

"It's good to have shadows
That run when you run
That laugh when you're happy
And hum when you hum
For you only have shadows
when your life's filled with sun."

The Drinks Are On Me

Foreword

This is the story of my family's breastfeeding journey, and then some. It explores a holistic approach to a subject little understood by the majority of people. Many professionals directly impact on a woman's choice to breastfeed. Despite their 'expertise', many doctors, midwives and health visitors know very little about breastfeeding, and unfortunately, pass on much misinformation.

I've learned that a successful breastfeeding story comes down to two things ~ education and determination. They go hand in hand. I recognise that if I'd not had the information, acted as a witness to living breastfeeding examples, or had access to support, my story and my parenting path would now read completely differently.

In an ideal world, your mother would have taught you everything about breastfeeding. You'd have learnt that when a baby is born, her mother's milk contains everything a growing brain and body need. Sadly, we don't live in an ideal world, and many mothers have been cut off from their inner knowing. The intuitive understanding of breastfeeding, which has been passed down through the ages, has been pushed aside by cultural shifts, the commercialisation of fake milk, and the destruction of the extended family. Many women have lost contact with the mothers and wise crones who could have shared the information contained in this book. The common knowledge has become uncommon.

By breastfeeding our babies, we pass this ancient knowledge and intuitive awareness onto our children at a deep cellular level where words and books are not needed. For the first time in our history, we are on the verge of breastfeeding dying out. When humans cease breastfeeding, the species will become extinct.

I'm not your mother, but I hope to give you the breastfeeding support a mother *could* have given, if she'd had it herself; so pull up a chair and enjoy, because, the drinks are on me!

Veronika Sophia Robinson
Eden Valley, Cumbria, UK
Autumn 2007

My favourite mammaries

Little lips puckering in anticipation of my breast, knowing that I'd read their cue and that my baby didn't have to cry or scream for a feed.

Moonlight shining on velvet-soft, newborn hair, as my baby and I snuggled closer in the night.

Of Eliza, aged six months, pushing Bethany off the neighbouring breast and jubilantly claiming it as her own.

Milk sprays ~ just like the Goddess Hera ~ truly a proclamation of abundance.

Waking to a voice asking "Do the boobas love me? Will they love me forever?"

Being asked before sunrise, "What are your breasts thinking about?"

Hearing my two year old at Christmas, singing *"Little Lord Jesus, no crying he makes, because his mama gives him booba."* Ah, bless!!

Waking up one morning to Eliza's hands feeling their way around my breasts, and her asking why there was a space in between. "There should be another boob in there."

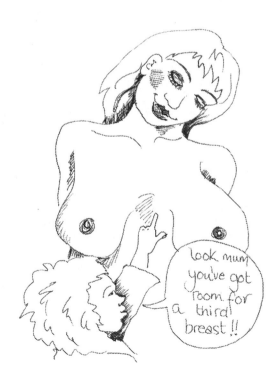

The Drinks Are On Me

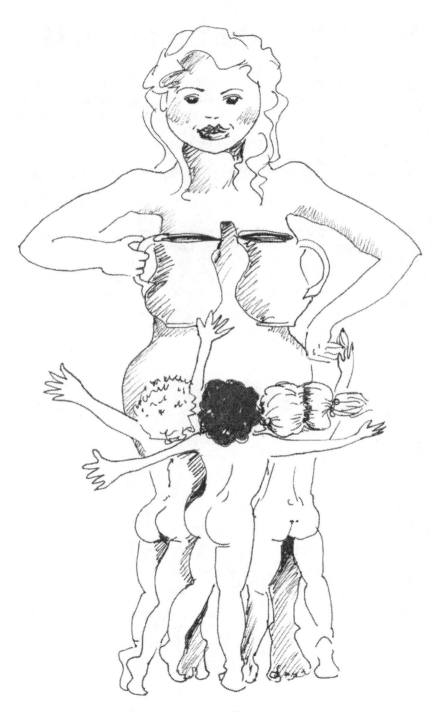

The Drinks Are On Me

Jugs
My story

Twenty years ago I was the sort of girl who'd walk into my local Aussie pub after work and say to my mates, "The drinks are on me!" High heels, make-up and short skirts defined me; my life revolved around having fun.

Despite being a late-blooming, flat-chested girl throughout secondary school, by the time I could 'shout drinks' at the pub, my male friends called me Jugs. In a few short years I'd well and truly busted out of my chest.

In my late teens and early twenties, I was your average 9 to 5 worker having a great time. Fun, back then, meant drinking late, lots of dancing till the wee hours, and weekend sleep-ins. With not a care in the world, and no-one depending on me, I could go off camping in the Australian bush at a moment's notice, and I often did.

Could anyone have accurately predicted the journey ahead of me, and how my jugs and free drinks would give way to a quiet, practical spirituality and eventually notoriety as an *extraordinary breastfeeder* in the UK and beyond? We don't walk through life alone. There are many people who influence our choices in life ~ and everything is a choice. Our journey is like a jigsaw puzzle, with pieces coming together, and the present moment fated by earlier decisions. Books, word of mouth, expertise, advice down the maternal lineage ~ they all paint a picture in our mind. When we arrive at choice points, very few people pioneer a new direction, instead repeating history in one form or another.

So what leads a woman to breastfeed her children for seven years apiece? Let me declare: I'm not a fruit cake, barking mad, or a space cadet for allowing my children to self-wean when they were ready. I can't have been dropped off from Planet X, because I've got the same little upturned nose as my mum, and I inherited my dad's small bum, which is totally inadequate for filling out jeans nicely! My mum, however, *might* be from another planet...but that's a whole different story and it's hers to tell.

This book exists to show that any woman with breasts can breastfeed her children as nature intended. I hope that by sharing my story, mothers around the world will feel that they can push back their culture's taboos and do what is right for their family. My story, and my family's journey, is based on intuition, as well as anthropological, biological, psychological research and studies, and ancient spiritual insights.

What makes my path to full-term breastfeeding different from many mothers in western culture is my compulsion to question absolutely everything. It's this questioning, this deep curiosity to look beyond standard, accepted norms, which has changed my life from party girl to ways completely unimagined.

When we choose to breastfeed our children, we take into the journey our own experiences of feeding in infancy. Although we may not consciously remember our early days, our body never forgets. As pre-verbal beings, we assimilated experiences received through our senses, and held the memory within every cell of our being. *The body never forgets.* Were we welcomed to our mother's breast? Did she willingly nourish us from her own body? Did she choose instead to feed us cow's milk or goat's milk? Were we abruptly weaned? Perhaps mother led us gently to foods in our second or third year of life. We may have breastfed until our needs were met. Regardless of the situation, the memory plays a part in how we choose to feed our children.

I was breastfed. My mother thinks it was for about six months, but hey, better to have your thirst quenched a little than to go through life parched, wondering why the elixir of life you were genetically promised, disappeared into thin air. Knowing everything I do about breastfeeding, I'm so very grateful my mother chose to breastfeed me.

She breastfed all eight of her children, the longest time being for about nine months. With four siblings younger than me, I had the benefit of seeing it as a normal, natural part of our everyday family life. They say a picture paints a thousand words. When we have breastfeeding depicted as the norm, the template of Nature's intention is printed indelibly in our subconscious, to be put to use some time in the future.

My family moved from Brisbane in Queensland, Australia, when I was six years old, away from the city to 700 acres in Freestone, on the Darling Downs. After a succession of farm failures due to drought (calves and crops dying), my dad moved into horse breeding. The dozens of horses, which were part of my idyllic childhood, played out their mammalian instincts year after year. Looking back, I was blessed to watch foals born before my very eyes; to watch mares having their period, and to watch one nursing mare adopt a newborn foal, and let it suckle, because its mother had died in birth. These stories fill the *mammary* banks of my mind, and confirm the miracle of what it means to be a mammal, regardless of our species. And though I wore school uniforms, and later danced till dawn in mini skirts, I, too, was a mammal, with instincts which would nurture my young.

Living on land, we had ample room for cats, which seemed to breed all the time. I loved to watch them give birth. They'd hide under my blankets to birth in the dark. I felt such excitement at watching the kittens nursing. It was here I learnt that mother mammals set limits. Mother cat would pat a kitten that was being too rough. We do this with our infants when they start to bite us at the breast. We say "no". And they learn very quickly, if they want more, to keep their teeth away.

My youngest three siblings were birthed at home. My mother deliberately chose to birth unassisted by doctor or midwife, an act which showed my young mind what it means to be a woman: to give birth naturally like our mammalian relatives, quietly, calmly and without an audience.

I reckon life's just one huge jigsaw puzzle, but often we don't get to see the complete, or even part of our 'destined' picture, till much later on down the track. My path to motherhood has been rich and varied, yet, funnily enough, sometimes the pieces came in ways I would never have imagined, and certainly didn't understand or appreciate at the time.

As a child, my mum used to talk about Montessori schools, and how they had child-sized furniture and made the classrooms especially suited to the children. The teacher didn't have a desk or stand at the front of the class, but instead was part of the classroom, acting as a guide, rather than an authority figure. When I was 16, I left Queensland and moved to the Adelaide Hills in South Australia. I was so thrilled to have escaped school, so it was all a bit of a shock to step off the Greyhound bus, after a day-long journey across deserts, to be greeted by my older sister, Heidi, who said that if I planned to live with her I had to go the local High School. How could she be so cruel?

Heathfield High School was near to The Children's Cottage, a small Montessori pre-school, run by former Mrs South Australia, Corraine Sopru. I loved this lady. She had a quiet spirituality, yet a dynamic personality. She was beautiful in every way imaginable. The Children's Cottage was run from the bottom of her garden in a converted building. Everything there was beautiful. The children's tables had miniature crystal vases on each one, and the children would go outside in the garden with tiny scissors, and little wicker baskets, to collect flowers.

I came initially for work experience during High School, and then voluntarily. Later on, I would become employed at the Hills Montessori School, not far away, as a teacher's aide. Before that though, I worked as a nanny for a middle-class family, looking after their two young daughters; and also for an Irish family with two adorable sons. I loved the children as if they were my own. Each night my heart would be torn in shreds when one of the little girls screamed for me as I drove away. Our bond was strong. At 19, I learnt how important it is for a young child to spend childhood with her mother as the main caregiver. At the Hills Montessori School, I worked helping all the children, and specifically an amazing boy called Sam, who had Down's Syndrome. Sam had *character*. He had a smile that could melt anyone's heart. Sam always had a snotty nose, but somehow it was easy to look past the bubbly, green gunk, because the light which emanated from his true being shone through so brightly. He would often climb onto the school roof and stand there smiling and laughing, while we all died a thousand deaths wondering how the heck he'd got up there, again. Sam took away my fear of Down's, and I knew that if I ever had a child with Down's Syndrome I'd love that child as much as I loved Sam.

His mum taught me a huge amount about the unconditional love of mothering. Some mothers choose to abort so-called 'faulty' babies, and other mothers allow their heart to be cracked wide-open and dare to love. Whose life is richer for the choices made?

The Drinks Are On Me

Although I was childless, I learnt so much about children and their needs, while I worked there. I saw first hand how asking a mother *not to* give her child white bread, packed with hundreds and thousands (coloured, sugary sprinkly things) and red cordial for lunch, made all the difference to the behaviour levels of a child. Overnight, the class hell-raiser became an incredibly lovely and charming individual. He was like that all along, it just got hidden while his brain was on overload. E-numbers, colouring and additives play havoc with the sensitive human brain, and yet a diet like this is commonplace in our society.

I witnessed how children are impressed upon so early by the values of their parents. To hear a four year old routinely say the 'f' word when failing to accomplish a chosen task, had me feeling like an old prude. Witnessing the pure beauty of a girl born with one leg, and the strength of spirit of a tiny girl with a growth disorder, showed me a human can overcome many, many things.

The school, at the time, was based in an old sandstone church. I loved working there ~ I loved the children, the teachers and the parents.

For some reason I will never understand, I was lured away from this idyllic job to become an office worker in an insurance company owned by one of the school children's dads. Well, I lasted a few weeks, and then decided to move back 'home' to Queensland.

Initially, I worked at the local special education unit. It was only part-time and didn't pay the bills, so I left for full-time work at the local hospital as a medical laboratory assistant. I feel sick to this day about some aspects of that job, including doing heel pricks on babies. It was nothing short of horrendous.

My boss left to travel overseas, and in came a man who would end up making my life hell, through sexual harassment. While talking with the hospital human resources manager, she asked me what sort of work I'd like to do. I told her of my love of writing, and she asked if I'd approached the local newspaper. Nope, hadn't done anything that obvious.

I phoned the editor of the Warwick Daily News, and he suggested I come down for a chat. He put me on 'emergency rounds' in the evenings, after I finished my hospital job. And by the end of the week, he'd thrown me completely in the deep end by sending me out reporting and photographing my own stories. It's ironic that my first front page story was about the wife of my former employer at the special education centre!

Even within the confines and restrictions of a newspaper 'house' style, my mum said that she could always tell my articles, as they were 'different' from the others. Perhaps the signs were already there that the writing I'd end up doing would be a step or five away from the mainstream.

I travelled to New Zealand at 23, and did bits of holiday work, before landing a fabulous job with the Royal New Zealand Society for the Protection of Animals. As their national media officer, I liaised with press all over the country, put together a book on the Society's history, and edited the children's section of their magazine.

In hindsight, I can see how all these projects would benefit my life down the track. The contract was for a year; then I travelled to the UK. While living in Hampshire I had a dream that I'd write a book on gentle birth. Never have I felt such a powerful dream. The words spoken to me were as real as anything I've ever experienced. Confused, as I didn't even want children and I didn't have a partner, I went into a local New Age bookstore, and two books on waterbirth literally fell off the shelf! No, really, they <u>did</u> fall.

I took them back to my studio apartment and devoured them. Something was rapidly changing within me. This was such a beautiful and gentle way to bring children into the world. Why weren't women everywhere doing this? Seeds were planted in my mind that would germinate a lot quicker than I could ever have imagined.

Back in New Zealand I experienced *pre-conception communication with my first daughter, who told me she'd be with me soon. "Hmmmm, so, er, who's the father?" Within weeks my soul mate turned up. My desire for a child by this point had become all-consuming. I met my husband, Paul, while working as an assistant to a Minister of Metaphysics, at an organisation where I'd also led workshops and courses in personal growth.

My pregnancy with Bethany ignited a passion for mothering which is still there to this day. Paul, my midwife Ruth Davison and I, founded the National Waterbirth Trust in New Zealand, to bring support, advice and resources to women seeking information on birthing in water. Paul and I also created the Peaceful Pregnancy cd, with affirmations and relaxing music. During pregnancy, I decided to become a nanny again. An overwhelming need to be with children before becoming a mother led me to Belinda and her daughter Imogen.

Belinda was a couturier, and taught at the local fashion college. Imogen was divinely beautiful, as blonde as it's possible to be, with a mass of curls. I carried her everywhere in a sling, even though I was heavily pregnant. Belinda would express breast milk for me to give Imogen during the day. Each lunch time I'd take her to Belinda's work so she could feed at the breast.

After I became a mum I went back to visit them. Standing on Belinda's verandah, chatting, Imogen became impatient with us and started screaming down the town. "Boobie. I want boobie now!" I laughed to hear her demand that her mum lie down on the verandah. Her behaviour seemed shocking at the time, but hindsight is such an enlightener. Not to mention a humbler.

Pre-conception communication has been experienced by many women, siblings and grandparents the world over. It is a conscious connection with the soul of an unborn child prior to its conception. A wonderful introduction to this topic can be found in the book, Soul Trek, by Elisabeth Hallett ~ see: www.light-hearts.com. It contains many beautiful stories of this communication. Women of adopted children have also had the experience of connecting with the soul of an unborn child who was destined for their family.

The Drinks Are On Me

We never know what life has in store for us, so judgements should always be made with caution, though preferably not at all.

Once, when I was having a bath with Imogen, she spied my naked breasts and pounced on me, latching herself on my breast. I was shocked, to say the least.

I usually looked after Imogen in her own home, but occasionally she'd come to our place. One time she'd had some left-over mashed avocado. I'd put it on the bench. My husband, being the usual clearer of all things left-over, promptly ate it. Perhaps he'd have not been so quick if I'd told him that Belinda's breast milk was used to thin it out! From that day on, he considered himself related to Belinda.

She provided me with a great example of attachment parenting, even though she worked outside the home. She practised attachment parenting by letting her child sleep in the family bed, breastfeeding beyond the standard six months and feeding her family organic wholefoods. She didn't vaccinate, and used a sling to provide body contact with Imogen so she could fully experience the 'in-arms' phase.

The main thing I've learnt from my journey through life, is the recognition that whatever we do, it *all* has meaning, no matter how mundane. In high school, the typing teacher used to hit my knuckles because I had an obsession with looking at the keyboard. Then she got all narky on me and put a bib over the keyboard so I couldn't see it at all. Needless to say, I quit that class. But Life wanted me to learn to type, and eventually I did. When I worked at the Warwick Daily News, I didn't have time to look at the keyboard. Typing is an invaluable skill which makes my writing life so easy because I can type as quickly as I think. Lightning fingers! All our experiences are valid. We should never underestimate how they'll contribute to our own mothering.

Learning how to breastfeed

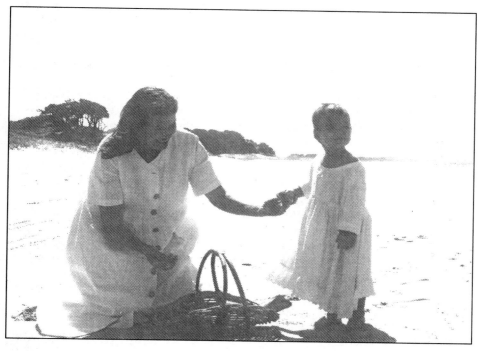

Collecting seashells with Bethany, Pakiri Beach, NZ

Now I lay me down to rest
Warm and safe near mother's breast
If I should wake before the dawn
I know that she will latch me on

Now I lay me down to rest
My precious baby by my breast
If she shall wake before the dawn
I'll hold her close and latch her on

(author unknown)

We live in a culture where the sight of a breastfeeding woman is not common. Indeed, she should be classed as a 'protected species'. Because we don't see it in our day to day life, we have to learn it when we become mothers. It's a skill which takes practice as well as commitment. Although the baby is born with a sucking reflex, he too is learning a new skill. Mother and child have to be patient. A positive mindset is the most important attitude we can bring to the breastfeeding relationship. Knowing that Mother Nature was aware of what she was doing when she created breasts, gives us faith that our body has everything it needs to feed our baby.

When we hear women say they 'couldn't breastfeed' it puts into our mind the possibility that our body might let us down. We do each other a disservice by perpetuating the myth that some women can't make milk.

Towards the end of your pregnancy you'll notice that your breasts are growing much larger. You might even notice some dried colostrum on your nipple, or some leaking. This is normal.

After you've given birth to your baby and the placenta, hormones will change in your body. Oestrogen and progesterone, which have been high during pregnancy, will now give way to prolactin. This hormone is responsible for 'bringing your milk in'.

Your baby's suckling sends messages from the nipple to your brain that the breast needs more milk. In response, you create more milk for your baby's next feed. **It's important to note that the breasts are never really 'empty' while you're lactating.** The term empty is used to describe a breast that's not *full* with milk.

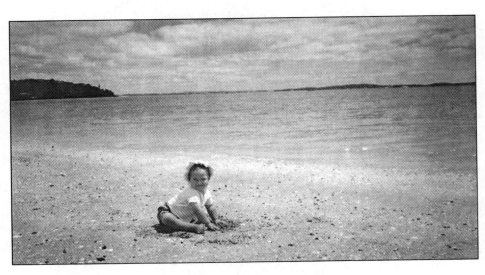

Bethany at 12 months of age and thriving on breast milk.

The Drinks Are On Me

Three Types of Milk

Colostrum
Foremilk
Hindmilk

There are three types of milk you'll make as a mother. Initially, there is colostrum for the first few days of your baby's life. From then on you make foremilk, which is thin and serves to satisfy thirst; and near the end of each feed is rich hindmilk. This satisfies hunger. Both foremilk and hindmilk are important at each breastfeeding session, so try not to think that your child only needs one or the other at any particular time.

During breastfeeding, two hormones are busy at work. Prolactin is producing milk, and oxytocin (the love hormone) is sending the message to bring down hindmilk. Some women have a distinct feeling in their breasts, known as letting-down, when this occurs. It can be experienced as a tingling sensation. The same hormones used in lovemaking are used in breastfeeding too. It's not unusual for some women to feel this sensation genitally as well. It's absolutely nothing to be ashamed of, or to feel uncomfortable about. It's **normal**. It's *completely* normal.

If you've been absent from your baby and are thinking about her, you might find the let-down sensation occurring. Many women find their breasts leak or spray milk as soon as they think of their baby, or even see or hear someone else's baby. This is natural. If you're in public and don't want your breasts to leak, you can press your hand or wrist (to be subtle) against your nipple for a few seconds or longer. Most women find this helps.

Successful breastfeeding depends largely on being relaxed. The more you breastfeed, the more relaxed you'll feel as oxytocin runs through your blood. Consciously create an environment where you know you can be yourself: a place where the only job to think about is breastfeeding your baby.

Holding a breastfeeding baby is a different experience for every woman. Some find it easiest to lie down on one side, in bed. Others need an armchair or rocking chair. Try to keep your neck relaxed while breastfeeding. The more you do it, the more confident you'll feel with various positions. To start with, however, make life as easy for yourself as possible. Save the fancy manoeuvres for when you really need them, like in a shop at the check-out, or placating a toddler with a bruised knee while you're on a business call, jotting down messages!

My own breasts were always full of milk (in the early months), and I found it easiest lying down. Both my daughters were often inundated with flowing milk, and it was helpful when they were a bit bigger, to lie flat on my back and let them 'work' for the milk, rather than have gravity pour it out for them.

The Drinks Are On Me

The importance of correct latching-on can not be overestimated in the aim of achieving pleasurable and successful breastfeeding. If you've got large breasts you'll almost certainly need to support your breast with one or both hands while your newborn gets used to feeding. Your job is to make it all as easy as possible. You can cup your breast with one hand while using your other to help support the baby's head. Baby's mouth needs to be fully open, so he can cover as much of your areola (large pink circle around your nipple) as possible. When ensuring correct latch-on, see that your baby is able to move her neck. When supporting her head, she must have neck freedom. Don't, under any circumstance, let your baby attempt breastfeeding by sucking only on your nipple, or with it only partly in her mouth. Three things will happen if you let this continue.

You'll end up with sore nipples and won't want to breastfeed.
Your baby will develop habits which don't serve her in the best way.
Your body won't get the message to let more milk down.

Always bring your baby *to* the breast, rather than take the breast to the baby. Your baby needs to be belly to belly with you.

Allow breastfeeding to be a peaceful time for both of you. Relax, breathe, just be there.

Babies learn to get used to the flow of milk coming out of your breasts. Initially you may have to help her, but allow your baby to be upright occasionally, and to take a rest from the breast if the flow is in full force.

Your baby is unique. Don't compare her feeds with another baby. Some need to feed for half an hour or more, while others are all done in ten minutes. Above all, *never* rush breastfeeding. Think about how you feel when you're running late for a meeting and you gulp down your food. It's not pleasant. Your baby doesn't understand rushing, so please, always plan your life around breastfeeding, not the other way around.

Honouring your baby's breastfeeding style will ensure that he is happy, content and feels secure and confident that his needs are being met by your perfectly attuned milk supply.

There is a reason you have two breasts. And it's got nothing to do with the chance of having twins or because men have two hands! By breastfeeding on two breasts, your babe learns to develop hand and eye co-ordination on both his right and left side.

It's not always necessary to breastfeed from both breasts at each sitting. Each breast can be alternated throughout the day and night. If you forget which side you fed from last, you usually only have to 'feel' the difference. One side will feel soft and empty, the other hard and full.

Developing a rhythm helps to establish breastfeeding for both of you. It can take about two months to feel really comfortable with breastfeeding, but some mums take longer, and this is perfectly normal.

Babies change so quickly, and just when we think we've a rhythm developed, something comes along to make us feel like we're complete beginners! Understandably, a woman can feel very vulnerable about breastfeeding and satisfying her baby's needs during these times.

Usually, by six weeks of age, you'll notice your baby going through a growth spurt and wanting to feed *all* the time. This will happen throughout the year, usually at six weeks, three, six and nine months ~ though bear in mind, every baby is different, so don't look to the calendar. And don't be fooled into thinking you're not making enough milk. If you let your baby breastfeed on cue, you'll **always** make enough milk.

Burping the baby

If we look to indigenous peoples, we find that they don't have the custom of burping the baby like we do in western culture. The reason for this is that their babies are almost always held upright and carried in slings. They also don't bottle-feed, a common cause of excess air being consumed with milk. It isn't necessary for a baby to be forced to burp after a feed. Discomfort usually comes from lying baby down after feeding.

Reflux

A holistic approach to reflux, where the baby ejects its milk, is to try and avoid him gulping air during feeds. Correct nipple latch, as always, is very important. Reflux is often defined as something experienced by a baby who is in pain and not gaining weight. This also usually includes an inability to breathe properly. It's best to avoid invasive tests, and choose a caregiver who can make a diagnosis from your baby's symptoms. Breastfeeding is actually the <u>best</u> way of treating reflux, provided the baby isn't having to deal with too much milk at once. (A study in 1995 showed that a mother's milk supply can be reduced through breastfeeding management).

As with colic, aim to keep your baby in an upright position as much as possible. Invest in a great sling. At all costs, don't lie down to breastfeed. Reflux is most commonly seen with formula milk-fed babies, and breastfeeding mums who have large amounts of caffeine and/or dairy in their diet.

The Drinks Are On Me

Saggy breasts!

Near the end of my pregnancy with Bethany, I was in the bath one night and observed just how much bigger my breasts had become. They were huge. I really didn't need this. Jugs are one thing, pitchers are a completely different story! I'd bought a bunch of gorgeously soft maternity bras which I managed to stretch completely out of shape before I even *started* breast-feeding. Not good. As I lay in the bath I noticed some dried milk around my nipple. Move over Archimedes. This was *my* eureka moment! Wow! My baby wasn't even born, yet I was capable of feeding her already. How miraculous.

A surprising number of women choose not to breastfeed because they fear having pendulous breasts. One person wrote on an internet forum, after seeing me on a breastfeeding documentary, that my breasts were 'dog-eared'. Hmmmppph! They were like that before I ever started breastfeeding.

A little known secret, but **please** shout it out to those far and near if it means we'll increase breastfeeding rates: breastfeeding *doesn't* wreck your breasts, pregnancy does. So if you want to avoid breast changes and pretend you're a teenage girl forever, either don't have a baby, or adopt a child instead.

Our breasts increase in size and change dramatically throughout pregnancy, but as it happens over the course of about seven months we lose sight of this fact, especially since they don't reduce in size again for a few months into breastfeeding (or years, in my case). Some women choose not to breastfeed, because they want to keep their breasts upright and perky. I can promise you 100% that breastfeeding doesn't make your boobs sag, pregnancy does.

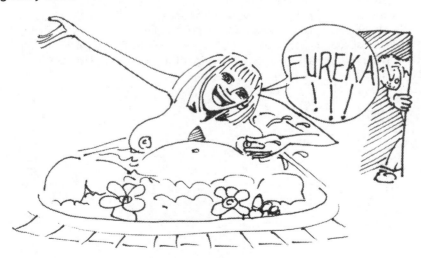

Biology class

I failed science throughout school. At least I'm consistent. They could have given me an A+ for that! I truly hated science class, and if Warwick State High School kept a log of sick room attendances, there'd be a very high chance that my visits <u>always</u> coincided with double biology lessons. If I wasn't in the sick room, I'd be up town. God love my biology teacher. He took me aside quietly one day and said that if I was going to keep wagging classes, to make sure I at least turned up first thing in the day, and at day's end, to register as present. Thanks mate! You're probably dead by now, but I just want to say I've learnt more about the mammalian aspect of human biology from being a passionate mum than I could ever have learnt in biol. class. And I'll bet *you* didn't know squat about breast milk.

As for chopping up frogs, it never did sit well with my vegetarian instincts! And let's face it, not even a butcher needs to know how to chop up frogs. Here's Veronika's primer on the biology of breastfeeding ~ made simple. Not *Breastfeeding for Dummies* as my husband suggested. Anyway, I'll comment on dummies later.

Breast milk is a cross between milk and blood.
It contains:

Carbohydrates
Proteins
Fats
Chloride
Macronutrients
Calcium
Minerals
Magnesium
Phosphorus
Potassium
Chromium
Copper
Fluoride
Iodine
Iron
Manganese
Molybdenum
Selenium
Zinc
Vitamin A
Vitamin B6
Vitamin B12
Vitamin C
Vitamin D
Vitamin E
Vitamin K
Biotin
Folate
Niacin
Pantothenic acid
Riboflavin
Thiamin

The Drinks Are On Me

Catalase
Histaminase
Arysulfatase
Antioxidants
a-Tocopherol
Cysteine
Ascorbic acid
Antiproteases a-l-antitrypsin
A-l-antiochymotrypsin
Prostaglandins
PG -E2; PG-F2
Secretroy IgA
Full antibody repertoire
Lysozyme
Lactoferrin
Interleukin-6
PAF-acetylhdrolase

Memory T CEs
EGF
NGF
Insulin
IGF-1
IGF -11
Relaxin
TGF-a
PRL
Corticosterone
TGF-b
GnRH
GRH
PTHrP
Peptides
Erythropoietin

Furthermore, these ingredients are made to a unique recipe for each baby, by its mother; and breast milk is different at **each** feed depending on the infant's age and stage-specific needs. A baby at one day old has different milk needs than one at three weeks old, for example, or a six month old baby. Your body knows the age of your baby and what stage she is at, and <u>exactly</u> what is needed in her breast milk every time she feeds. It can not be duplicated in any way, shape or form. Not even by the same mother at a different time of day! How groovy is that? And people wonder why breast-feeding advocates get all excited!

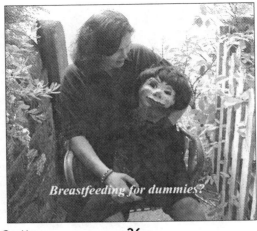

Breastfeeding for dummies?

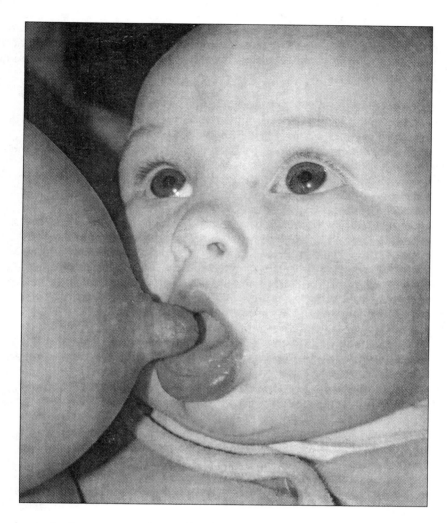

Andorra preparing to latch-on.

The Drinks Are On Me

Formerly undiscovered ingredients in breast milk are being found all the time. We only know the tip of the iceberg. One hundred years from now we'll still be discovering more about its amazing properties. People often wonder if there's enough iron in breast milk for a baby, and mistakenly start offering solid foods. The iron in breast milk is able to be assimilated by the baby, and is always 'enough'. Easy facts that anyone can remember (if they want to, that is).

Breastfeeding helps your uterus go back to its normal size.
Skin-to-skin contact creates a strong bond between mother and child, with an increased sense of security and comfort.
Breastfeeding builds the immune system, which doesn't mature till about seven years of age.
A decrease in ovarian and uterine cancers in women who breastfeed has been proven in many studies.
Breast milk kills polio/meningitis.
Breast milk is easily digested, and provides, in just the right proportions, the essential nutrients, vitamins, proteins, fats and antibodies that the baby needs to develop physically and neurologically. More and more research is showing that breastfeeding leads to optimal brain development. Breast milk contains over 200 immunological agents that cannot be replicated by science. Research shows breastfeeding also helps protect the baby against allergies and reduces the rate of serious illness.
Breastfeeding decreases the risk of tooth decay.
Breastfeeding is free! Even if a baby is drinking expressed breast milk and you need to purchase feeding accessories, it will be far less than what you would spend on formula.
Breastfeeding decreases a mother's chances of developing breast cancer. This benefit is strongly connected with the length of your breastfeeding experience.
Breastfeeding helps the baby to develop right and left hand-eye co-ordination (ideally we change our baby from one breast to the other for alternate feeds).
Breastfeeding may actually result in stronger bones and reduced risk of osteoporosis. Studies show that after weaning her children, a breastfeeding mother's bone density returns to pre-pregnancy levels or even higher.
Breastfeeding develops the oro-facial muscles.
Breastfeeding mothers show less anxiety and depression postpartum than formula-feeding mothers, because breastfeeding triggers and releases oxytocin (sometimes called the love hormone), that can help you relax and feel less stressed.
You'll burn extra calories, aiding weight loss. Milk production burns 200 to 500 calories a day.
Breastfeeding saves time. ([52]All of the above studies/statements can be found in research/published medical studies held by La Leche League International)

How mother's milk is made

Breast milk is made in the alveoli ~ large numbers of sac-like structures, and taken to the nipple via milk ducts. A nipple is sensitive, because of the numbers of nerves it contains. The large round circle surrounding the nipple, called the areola, contains glands which emit oil. This helps to maintain good nipple health.

The milk-secretion reflex involves the baby sucking at the breast, which in turn sends a message to the pituitary gland, which then produces prolactin. This then sends a message to 'make milk'. At the same time, the infant's sucking causes the pituitary gland to send oxytocin, the love hormone, into the blood. Once this message arrives in the breasts, the milk lets down. This is commonly known as the let-down reflex.

The emptier the breast is, the faster it tries to refill. (Remember, they're never *really* empty!). If milk is regularly and thoroughly removed from the breast, more will keep being produced. Exceptions to this might include when there is a retained placenta, contraceptive pills disrupting the hormones, or breast surgery. It might also be because the baby's being supplemented with formula, and therefore the mum's body is receiving the message that adequate milk is being made. If the baby isn't being given enough access to the breast throughout the day and night, and/or the breastfeeding session ends before the baby has had enough, problems with milk supply will occur. Likewise, if there is some sort of latch-on problem, the baby will not be removing enough milk, and again, the message won't get to the pituitary gland to produce more.

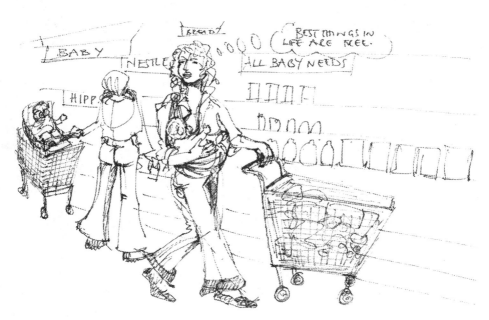

The Drinks Are On Me

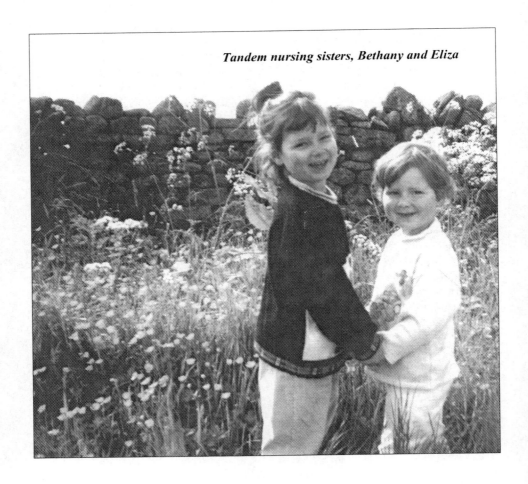

Tandem nursing sisters, Bethany and Eliza

"God gave me hands so I could hold mummy's BBs (breasts)"

Bethany Robinson, aged four.

Vitamin K

The routine injection of vitamin K into newborn babies is another example of mankind's inventions coming between mother and child. The purpose of artificial vitamin K is to prevent haemorrhagic disease of the newborn (HDN). We must always ask ourselves why any man-made intervention has been introduced.

How did humanity manage to exist for so long without vitamin K injections? What have we, as a species, done to mothers and babies that we consider it 'necessary' to have vitamin K? When a baby is born vaginally, without intervention, she takes in some of her mother's faeces on the way through the birth canal. This goes into her gut and initiates the development of the *immune system*. When birth became modernised, women were given enemas before birth, so babies no longer received the gut-enhancing faeces. Modern birth also means that breastfeeding is inevitably delayed, as birth-care professionals follow through on their various procedures ~ such as cleaning and weighing the baby. This delay in the baby receiving breast milk means she doesn't receive vitamin K **naturally** from her mother's milk.

Circumcision often meant babies bled to death. So, we intervene in birth, delay breastfeeding and chop off bits of our baby's body. Of course we'll need vitamin K!

A study showed that the risk of a baby who didn't get vitamin K, developing HDN, is somewhere between one in 10,000 and one in 25,000[57]. Babies who have gentle births are highly unlikely to develop HDN. Rarely, however, will the medical profession tell mothers of the link between intramuscular vitamin K and childhood cancer. There are alternatives to this. Be prepared, however, to hear that all babies are born with low vitamin K, and that breast milk is low in vitamin K. Mother Nature, *what was she thinking?*

As mothers who make informed choices, we need to ask ourselves to whom the level of a baby's vitamin K is being compared? Could it be that this low level is actually **normal** for a **baby**, just like it's normal for a baby to have a big head compared to its body[58]?

The babies who are most at risk are those born via medically managed births: those births we'd consider traumatic ~ caesarean, ventouse, forceps.

Studies declaring breast milk to be low in vitamin K were taken during a time when women used to express colostrum and not give it to their babies. These women also fed their babies on a schedule, and feeds were restricted, as was the amount of time spent on the breast. Common sense would tell you this is an unreliable way of studying vitamin K levels in breast milk. Colostrum, and hindmilk (produced near the end of a baby's feed), both contain vitamin K. If neither of these were likely to have been part of the study, then what sort of information are we passing on to women?

One of the best ways to support your baby's vitamin K levels is to allow the cord to remain uncut for as long as possible.

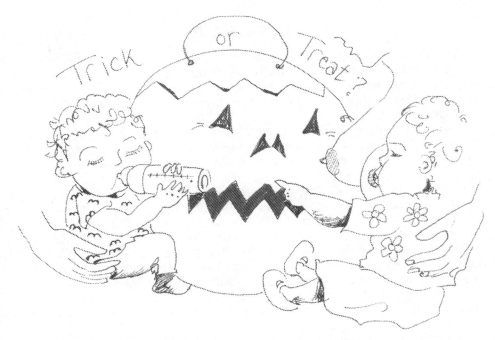

Some women choose a lotus birth, leaving the placenta and cord attached to the baby for a few days after birth, until the cord dries and breaks naturally. Even allowing the cord to stay uncut until your placenta delivers naturally (without drugs) helps enormously. Remember, cord blood belongs to **your baby**. Please don't give it away or let anyone steal it.

A maternal diet with vitamin K
Alfalfa sprouts
Seaweeds
Green leafy vegetables
Kelp
Lentils
Peas
Organic unsulphured blackstrap molasses

If you regularly include the above foods in your diet, you can rest assured your baby will get plenty of vitamin K from you, initially through the placenta, then from your breast milk.

Breastfeeding begins

One night in March, birth entered our home on tip-toes. Softly, quietly into the night, our daughter arrived. By candlelight, Bethany was birthed naturally, into the warm water of a birthing pool, beside our bed. I put her to my breast while we waited for the placenta to come out. In hindsight, I wish I'd had a chair in the birth pool, because buoyancy and big boobs don't make great companions: and I found it difficult to initiate breastfeeding in the pool. However, once Paul and I got into bed with Bethany, she fed beautifully.

Meconium ~ learning lessons from poo!

During the first 24 hours after Bethany's birth, it became apparent she'd swallowed some meconium because she vomited up some with her milk. Meconium is a fancy word for baby poo that's made in utero and looks like tar ~ black and sticky. Of all babies who release meconium at birth, less than ten percent appear to have done so because of distress. I have no reason to believe Bethany was distressed during birth.

We were blessed to have such a wise midwife as Ruth Davison. She suggested we keep breastfeeding Bethany, as the milk would dilute the meconium and make it easier to clean her stomach. Just about every other midwife would have panicked and sent us off to hospital for our baby to have a full stomach pump. It was one of our early lessons in listening to the body, and working with nature.

Bethany breastfed happily through infancy and toddlerhood, remaining a strong, healthy and happy child.

When she was a few months old we were visiting our friends Teresa and Marshall. Marshall asked me when I'd planned to finish breastfeeding. It stopped me in my tracks, as it was the first time I'd ever consciously thought about weaning.

"Maybe a year or so, whenever she's had enough I suppose," I answered. I really had never thought of ending the process; somehow it seemed irrelevant while I was nursing a young baby. Even back then I was aware that breastfeeding was no sacrifice, and would only involve a short amount of time in my life. How could I have even begun to imagine the direction my life would take as a result of this simple question? "When will you stop breastfeeding?"

The more baby feeds,
the more milk you'll make.

The Drinks Are On Me

Colostrum
Nature's liquid gold for babies

Colostrum, the thick, yellowish milk produced in the first few days after birth, is rich in nutrients and also helps the baby to pass meconium (first stools), as it is a laxative. Beats Epsom salts any day! It also helps prevent jaundice. Try to get your baby to the breast as soon as possible after birth.

Every mother with surgically undamaged breasts has <u>enough</u> milk. If you try to hand-express, it may seem as if you don't have much. *Supply and demand* means giving your baby the breast on cue. That is, **before** the baby cries, and at least every two hours, offering both breasts.

If you decide to formula-feed your baby, at the very least allow him to receive your colostrum for a few days, as it's so rich in nutrients and anti-bodies. Colostrum starts being produced during pregnancy. High in carbohydrates, antibodies and protein, low in fat, and highly concentrated in nutrients, it's very easy for your baby to digest.

To maximise your baby's intake of colostrum, it's important to encourage plenty of breastfeeding, say at least 10 - 12 sessions per day ~ more if you can. While this is happening, it allows the mature milk to start forming, and also helps you to avoid engorgement.

Although colostrum seems to come out as such a small amount, it's important to realise that for each baby-sized mouthful, there are **countless** numbers of living cells which will defend your baby against many harmful diseases. Consider it Nature's Immunisation Programme.

During pregnancy, your baby received an antibody called secretory immunoglobulin A (IgA), via the placenta. Your baby was protected from infections as a result. Now, colostrum will continue the job of protecting him. Another important role of first milk is to prevent attack in the baby's gastrointestinal tract by foreign foods and substances. Throughout the time your child breastfeeds, his immune system will benefit enormously from your milk, and protect him from diseases and viruses.

Please don't be scared that the amount of colostrum produced for your baby will leave him hungry. Babies aren't like adults. An adult's stomach is about the size of a clenched fist, yet most of us in western society continually eat three times as much as we can fit in there comfortably. Your baby's tummy is more like the size of a raspberry! Within a week, his stomach will expand to hold about twice that amount. All you need to think about is breastfeeding. Just trust that your baby is getting everything he needs. If you supplement with formula, or offer a dummy, you'll be reducing your milk supply, and also risk engorgement.

It's important that babies breastfeed from *both sides,* so they can develop correct eye and hand co-ordination. If you have difficulty getting comfortable, try different positions, such as lying down. Use cushions or blankets for support, if necessary.

Newborn babies should be encouraged to nurse at least ten to twelve times in a twenty four hour period. They should have one or two *really* wet nappies in this time. After the milk increases, expect six to eight really wet nappies and two to five bowel movements a day.

If your baby has lost over 7% of birth weight, and not regained it in a week or two, it's not necessarily that you're short of milk. It's more likely to be a case of breastfeeding mismanagement.

Check to see baby is attached properly, swallowing, and having wet nappies. One way to assess correct latch-on is to see how your nipples feel. Sore nipples are nearly always caused by improper latch-on. Imagine a tube of toothpaste and trying to get the toothpaste out by squeezing the hard part at the top. Now try and squeeze by putting your fingers on the tube. Breastfeeding employs the same idea. The baby's mouth needs to be right around the nipple and areola. Remember, it's not called nipple feeding.

> *Although colostrum seems to come out*
> *as such a small amount,*
> *it's important to realise*
> *that for each baby-sized mouthful,*
> *there are __countless__ numbers*
> *of living cells*
> *which will defend your baby*
> *against many harmful diseases.*

The Drinks Are On Me

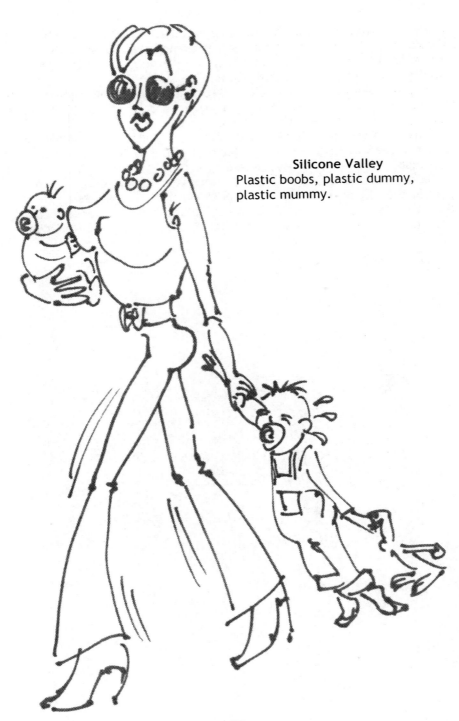

Silicone Valley
Plastic boobs, plastic dummy,
plastic mummy.

The Drinks Are On Me ~ 36 ~

Disconnected parenting

Young children are one with us, so we should stop seeing them separately, and wanting to separate from them when we feel they're too needy. There's no question that humans are incredibly creative, intelligent and ingenious. However, man-made devices designed to improve and simplify parenting, more often than not get in the way of wholesome mothering simply because we lose touch, literally, with our child.

Artificial milk

Fake milk disconnects mother and child in many ways. Mother's milk is made by her body, which scans the environment for pathogens, and then provides natural immunity to her child. This is a strong connector between mother and child. Artificial milk is incapable of doing this. It's a static product made in a laboratory. It has no recognition of pathogens and disease, and nor does it recognise one baby from another. No laboratory or scientist will ever be able to provide love in a liquid form for our babies.

Bottle-feeding

By receiving milk from a bottle, even breast milk, the baby or child doesn't receive the same comforters that come from feeding at the breast ~ a place where we hear our mother's heartbeat, tune into her breathing, feel comfort suckling, and are embraced in her arms. We're one with her when breastfeeding. Anyone can bottle-feed a child. Young babies are often left with bottles propped up against a pillow, denying them any human contact! When breastfeeding, a mother breathes in her babe's smell, and her breast milk adjusts to her baby's needs. If the baby has contact with bacteria or pathogens, the mother's milk adapts appropriately. Her body is always 'on guard' to protect her baby. This doesn't happen with bottle-fed babies, nor can the same adjustments take place with expressed milk, because it isn't fed to the baby at the time it was expressed.

Dummies

Dummies don't replace the love, warmth and attention of a mother. They stop the baby and child expressing their real needs. Just who is the dummy pacifying? See page 47.

Leash/rein/strap/harness

Our toddlers aren't dogs, they're children. Yes they can be busy and move quickly, but this is why, as mothers, we were given hands ~ to hold our children and provide warmth and comfort, and to be side by side with them while they talk about the environment they're exploring. This is another example of a clever device that removes us from our biological drive as parents.

The Drinks Are On Me

Cots/cradles

No other mammal sleeps apart from its young, so why do we? What makes humans so far removed from the biological needs of their young that they would consider such a barrier during sleep time? If this seems a leap for you, imagine what it would be like if you couldn't sleep with your partner each night? What if the only contact you had was for procreational sex, rather than recreational love-making, cuddles, laughs, heart to heart talks?

Imagine what it would be like to sleep in a different room to someone you love, night after night. Or if that person had to sleep behind bars, even in the same room. This is what many people do to their babies. Babies don't know why we do this! What they know *is* that every cell of their body is telling them to be with their mother.

Why aren't we listening? Why do we get so caught up in the colour of a nursery, the Peter Rabbit wall-paper, the musical toys designed to get our baby to sleep, and other people's opinions? Babies don't *need* any of this. Pretty nurseries, beautifully carved cradles and state of the art cots have only one purpose ~ to give parents physical space away from the baby. The needs of the baby are completely ignored.

Prams/buggies

A human spends approximately nine months in utero. The first nine months outside the womb are <u>also</u> a time of gestation, and we, as parents, are meant to carry our babies close to our chests, our hearts, our breath. While buggies can be immensely helpful for older children when they can't walk long distances, they are not suitable for meeting the needs of infants. When we sling our babies, from day one, we feel the familiar sense of connection right for our species. We only have to look to nature, or how we'd be parenting in nature, to see that our man-made devices are inhibitors to natural parenting.

Car seats

Car seats, apart from not accommodating the baby's natural body shape, do much damage to the spine. There was a time people used them simply for transporting a baby in the car. Nowadays people use them for carrying babies everywhere, even while asleep, and this is *not* good. It's one more invention that was created for parents, but not for babies. Clearly, most mothers in western culture rely on a car for travel. I urge you not to keep your baby in a car seat for a minute longer than necessary, even if it means disturbing them from sleep. Only use them for travel. If you have to travel in a car regularly, make it a priority for your child to have cranio-sacral therapy or chiropractic adjustments, on a regular basis.

Baby walkers

This isn't a natural way to walk. It's an artificial child-minder which has the potential to be very dangerous. Many, many accidents have happened as a result of baby walkers.

A child needs to experience crawling, and then learning to walk as a *vital* part of brain development. It's part of life to fall over when we take our initial steps. Baby walkers keep parents entertained and give them the freedom to be separated from their baby, in order to do other things. They don't help a baby learn to walk. Learning to walk comes from developing a sense of balance, falling over, getting up and trying again. It's a trial run for the rest of their life.

Baby monitors

A nice idea, in theory, for it's far better to be able to hear your baby if you're elsewhere, than not to hear them at all. However, we are meant to sleep with our babies. If you use one by day, then why aren't you sharing the room with your baby while she sleeps? A baby can sleep on a soft pillow safely on the floor, in any room of the house where you are, or sleep in a sling. If you rely on a baby monitor to know if your baby is awake or asleep, gurgling or screaming, vomiting, choking or breathing, then you're **too far away** from her.

Televisual stimulus

Where tv was once used as 'family entertainment', more and more parents are now relying on it to entertain their babies and children. In the US there is a station dedicated for children under 12 months of age! Using tv or a computer screen to provide entertainment to infants and toddlers short-circuits creativity, subjects a child to electromagnetic pollution and numbs the brain to a hypnotic state within one minute of screen viewing.

Wholesome mothering

We don't need man-made inventions for wholesome mothering. Listening to our baby is all we ever need to keep the relationship intact, and allow for his optimal development. We simply continue the ecstasy of conception, pregnancy and natural birthing into other areas of our life. If parents considered that <u>all</u> babies are born prematurely and are highly dependent, a new attitude to caring for infants would emerge. It takes nine months to grow a baby on the inside of our body, and gestation *continues* after birth ~ we do this optimally through breastfeeding on-cue, sharing sleep and sling wearing.

Crying babies

It used to be that when a baby was born, it would be hung upside down and its bottom smacked. The idea behind this barbaric thinking was to open their lungs and get circulation going. A gentle and conscious parent would, instead, massage the baby's skin. It has been proven that it's physiologically harmful for an infant to cry. This happens on many levels.

Firstly, it can cause hoarseness. It reduces blood oxygen levels, dramatically increases the heart rate, disturbs digestion and can lead to fainting. Crying drains a baby's energy.

The hormone cortisol floods the bloodstream. This negatively impacts on the developing brain. Other negative risks include distress in the respiratory system, breathing troubles, puncturing of the lungs, and intra-ventricular haemorrhage.

When we allow our baby to cry unnecessarily, we're teaching it negative socialisation skills. It's here that our infant learns that its caregiver doesn't, in actual fact, 'care'. As a parent, when we allow our child to cry without attending to their needs, we become detached emotionally. All the traumatic states mentioned lead to our child having a delayed psycho-social adaptation to life after birth.

Our baby, when left to cry, will make poor eye-contact after such distress, and may not breastfeed as effectively. He is, in essence, shutting down to the relationship with the caregiver.

Hard crying leads to poor learning, and affects sleep patterns. If you view a good cry as positive for your infant, then you're not realising that the sleep-induced state it brought on is, in fact, a response to *stress*. This is **not** healthy or safe. Be aware that this negatively affects your baby's organs and internal systems.

The purpose of a baby's cry is to alert her mother. Ideally, if she's in tune with her baby, she'd feel upset, and attend to her. This is a **normal**, natural and biologically designed response. It should make the mother's heart-rate and blood-pressure increase. Her nipples should become erect, and milk let-down will occur.

Crying is designed to alert a baby's mother to danger. In our culture there is far too much crying. An in-tune mother will not need her baby to cry. She'll see and hear her baby cue her for food, to pee or poo, or sleep. And she will respond by cuddling, or by changing the baby's position, by feeding or getting him to sleep.

At one extreme of parenting, we have a style which encourages complete distancing between parent and child. And at the other end, a style promoted to attachment parents under the idea that if you love your child, and stay near her, she can cry all she likes. Both styles are completely ignorant of, and out of touch with, an infant's needs. Both are based on a parent's desire, and not the child's needs.

While crying may be healing for *adults*, this doesn't mean it's the same for infants. Infants are non-verbal, and have not developed their other systems, whereas adults have.

Both approaches diminish the intuitive tie between mother and child. This leads to separation and does nothing to maintain bonding between them. It's passive, detached and creates emotional separation. As mammals, this is completely contrary to our biological evolution and needs. Studies have shown that this very act of emotional separation and detachment can lead to violence later on in life[56].

It is emotional neglect. When we do this to our children, we're teaching them, in a non-verbal way, that it's 'normal' and therefore 'right' to not feel the pain and hurt of other human beings.

We fool ourselves if we believe that not attending to the needs of a crying baby is any different than if we were to leave them crying in a room alone. Babies who are denied comfort through the breast will be deficient in tryptophan. Later on in life, they'll be more likely to suffer from depression.

An infant doesn't **want** to cry. It cries so that its mother will come and *stop* the crying. It's a **late** call to needs. Whatever the needs: comfort, heat, breast milk, suckling for comfort, the baby is calling *you* to relieve its problems. It <u>relies</u> on you. If this is so hard to understand, then try putting yourself into baby slippers for a minute or two. Imagine that you're screaming your lungs out and no one cares. What would this teach you about life, about love?

By forcing a baby to self-soothe we're inadvertently interfering with their skill development. They're compromised.

Our culture has a high rate of thumb sucking and the use of dummies and pacifiers. Cultures which allow babies to nurse on-cue have no incidence of thumb sucking. When we meet the needs of our infants, they'll have no need to suck fingers, thumbs, artificial objects or even more sadly, to bang their heads, self-rock, body-rock or head-roll. Most humans would be horrified to see these actions occurring in animals kept in captivity. Yet why do we ignore it in our own children?

It's so easy to recognise when our baby needs attention. We don't need to wait for her to cry. Look and listen to her fidgets, grimaces, fussing and agitation. This is her way of *communicating*. Some babies never need to cry. When we truly care for our baby, nurse on cue, rather than on demand, and carry the baby so they have sensory stimulation, they have very little reason to do so.

It can take just over a minute for the unmet needs of a baby to go from a small cry to a crying scream of pain. Quick and intuitive responses by a mother lead to a happy, contented baby.

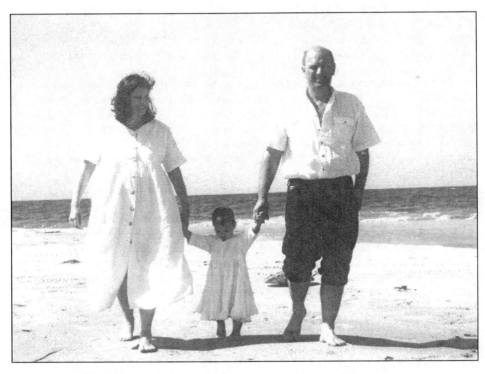

Pregnant with Eliza, Pakiri Beach, New Zealand

The manual for parenting

How often do we hear people say that there should be a manual for parenting? Nature *did* give us a manual! It's within every cell of our being, and our baby presents it to us. When we listen to our baby, the hormones and neurons work closely together to develop bonding. They can not be misinterpreted. They are loud, clear and concise. The only way you can't hear these messages is when you listen to someone other than your baby or inner self.

Moobs

MOOBS ~ otherwise known as Man Boobs, became rather famous when the then UK Prime Minister, Tony Blair, and Leader of the Conservatives, David Cameron, were photographed on their summer holidays, sporting a pair of baps in sizes many women would die for. And yes, it's true that men can lactate...

Men often say that they feel left out when it comes to breastfeeding, and this is then used as an excuse for babies to start receiving expressed breast milk or to be bottle-fed artificial milk. *Nobody* benefits from this, especially the baby. Let's get clear on a few things here. Girls, let men feel like the superior sex, ok? It's no skin off our nose. We don't need any badges or medals; and well, we know the truth (shhhh!), but here's the thing: whether a father feels left out because of breastfeeding, or feels like he's part of the parenting package, it all comes down to choice - that is, a bit of wiring in his head determining how he chooses to **see** breastfeeding. Explain it to your partner in electrical terms, it'll probably make sense. Meanwhile, I'll explain it in girly terms so you know what I'm ranting about, because it's very important that babies are fed from the breast rather than the bottle, if at all possible. Breastfeeding isn't just about milk.

Men can't grow babies in their bellies. But they can *massage* our bellies to give us support. They can love and talk to our babe in utero. Though men can lactate, simply because they too have mammary glands, they aren't designed to breastfeed. Let's look at why women are the breastfeeders ~ apart from the fact that most girls don't have hairy boobs!

Babies don't bond with dads through bottle-feeding. End of story. The bonding which occurs through breastfeeding is unique to that experience and can not be replicated with a bottle. Dads bond in other ways. It's a different and vital experience, not a lesser one. The greatest gift a father can give his partner and child is to support the mother in her breastfeeding relationship.

What our men can do for us, and our baby, is to protect, provide and nurture.

By feeding at their mother's breast as babies and young children, a child stabilises its body temperature, heart and breathing rates. If she is teething, or in any sort of discomfort, breastfeeding acts as a natural analgaesic. At the breast, she receives the correct live cells and antibodies that her mother's body has made by responding to the environment. It's only at the breast that she'll correctly develop the jaw and palate. The artificial nipples which are available can't come close to replicating a human nipple. They may 'seem' similar in shape, but there's no comparison in function, or in the way the baby suckles on it. When dad feeds babe breast milk from a bottle, she doesn't get the breastfeeding experience.

The Drinks Are On Me

The Monogamy Hormone

It's not just women who have hormones course through their blood in relation to parenting. Men do too. Vasopressin (also in women but to a much lesser degree) is a hormone which promotes strong paternal behaviour. This occurs when a man is living with his pregnant partner. Testosterone drives a man, encourages aggression and tempts him towards other women. Vasopressin tempers it by having the opposite effect. It encourages a father to be dedicated to his partner, protective, stable, and want to touch and be touched. It helps him bond with his baby.

The hormone is triggered through being near to the mother in pregnancy, and with the mother and child during and after birth. The ability of his body to interpret his partner's hormones is due to him detecting the change in her pheremones (steroid hormones on her skin). Clearly the closer he is to her physically, the stronger the reaction will be.

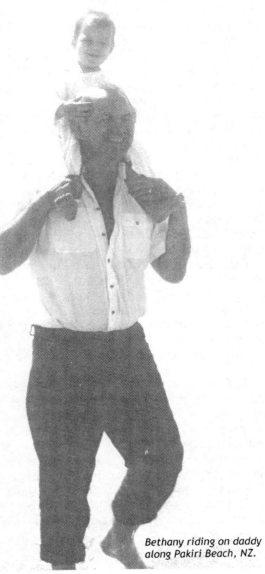

Bethany riding on daddy along Pakiri Beach, NZ.

Practical things dad can do for mum and baby

Feeling left out of the breastfeeding experience isn't about how a man's partner is relating to their baby, it's about how **his** mother related to **him**! When he can understand this, not only can healing occur, but he can create *new* patterns in parenting, which will benefit generations to come.

Some people decide to express milk so the father can be part of the nursing process. **It's far better for the baby to be <u>breastfeeding</u>.** Although breast milk in a bottle is unquestionably superior to formula milk, we mustn't fool ourselves. It doesn't *nourish* in the way breastfeeding from our mother's breast does.

The father's most important job in breastfeeding is to *enhance* the nursing relationship between mother and child. A baby has so much to gain from a father he gets to spend time with ~ a bond develops which will last a lifetime. The father becomes a role model for how males can express affection. The child also develops a healthy self-esteem. Author Steve Biddulph says that fathers who become engrossed with the baby are much more committed to their safety and care. "This seems to engage the protective instincts of a father, and he will be five times *less likely* ever to harm, or abuse a child."

There are plenty of ways for a father to be involved. These include:
putting baby in a sling and going for a walk
spending time with the other children
bringing the mother plenty of pure water, home-made vegetable soup, fresh fruit or vegetable juice, smoothies, herb teas
offering nutritious snacks
talking with mum
talking with baby
sleeping with baby
affirming what a wonderful job mum is doing breastfeeding and mothering
playing soft, gentle music or an instrument
stroking baby
having a bath with baby
screening visitors so mum and babe can rest
helping with housekeeping!
preparing food
soothing baby to sleep with a gentle back rub
singing to baby
learning about elimination communication (listening to the baby's cues to pee and poo, thereby eliminating the need for nappies)

The Drinks Are On Me

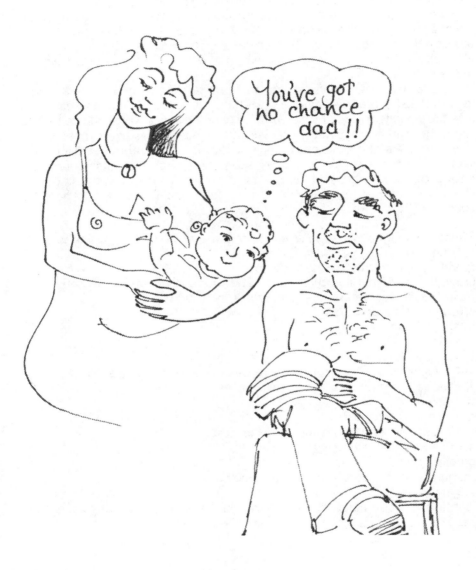

Who's the dummy?

When Eliza was born in New Zealand, staff in the hospital's Neonatal Intensive Care Unit (NICU) were worried she wouldn't be able to swallow, and kept trying to offer her a dummy. "NO!" I yelled. I rallied my mother to let Eliza nurse at her breasts (which had lovingly nurtured eight of her own children). The staff *wrongly* thought that Eliza had swallowed water during a waterbirth, and were treating her for a possible lung infection.

After three unbearable days of nil-by-mouth, the staff suggested formula down a tube for Eliza. "No" I said. Actually, I yelled "no". Nothing like a mother bear protecting her young by getting vocal. "Just a little bit?" they asked. "ROAR". They got the message. I expressed milk diligently, and watched like a hawk to make sure it was the only fluid going down the tube into Eliza's body. Why do parents have to fight for this? Hospital staff should be 100%, no questions asked, behind parents and their baby initiating exclusive breastfeeding. Every parent and Health Care Provider should fully understand the implications of *not* breastfeeding. When Eliza came to my breasts for the first time, still attached to loads of tubes and wires, she breastfed beautifully. The sucking reflex, that every child is born with, was able to be developed thanks to my mother's nipple, which matched my own far more accurately than the best dummy in the world ever could have. She also received the in-arms experience as soon as we were able to get her out of the incubator.

If you find yourself in hospital with a baby needing special care, etc., don't be coerced into believing an incubator is necessary for your baby. The two reasons babies are kept inside these plastic bubbles are to provide a regular temperature, and convenience for staff. It's vital for a parent to understand that cribs are for the **convenience** of the nursing staff. They are *not* designed for your baby's health and well-being.

Kangaroo care

Kangaroo care needs to be clearly defined. In hospitals they usually take it to mean a little cuddle here and there. Well, as an Australian girl born and bred, I know a thing or two about kangaroos, and one thing they **don't** do is kick their wee joey out of the pouch for most of the day! Kangaroo care is <u>24 hour a day skin-to-skin holding</u>[1]. When you do so, your baby's body temperature will be maintained. There is absolutely **no** reason why a child can't be treated in its parents' arms. The priority should be the well-being of the child, for whom skin-to-skin contact with a parent is <u>vital</u> for optimal growth. If you, as a parent, are committed to body contact (kangaroo care) and are prepared to hold the baby to your chest around the clock, then you can say goodbye to the incubator. As a parent, you can tell the doctor and nursing staff that your body contact will help to regulate your baby's heart beat, establish better breastfeeding, allow for better weight gain, etc.

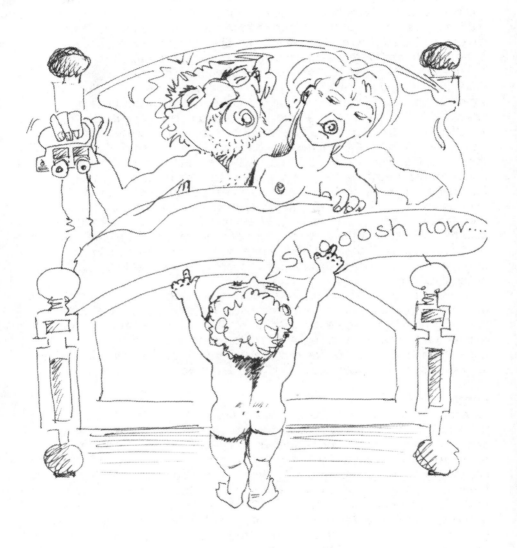

Statistically, babies separated from moth
getting breastfeeding established. I knew thi:
clock for each other while Eliza was banned f
tistics hadn't counted on my sheer determina
ing.

What happens when a baby has a dummy?

The term dummy has now, for the most pai
because people, frankly, don't want to be ren
the baby 'dumb'. Studies show reduced intellig
use. It's often given to those babies who are too   ...ummy
mouth and say what they're really wanting!   .. to pull it out of their

The only ones to benefit from a dummy are the parents, though separation from their child doesn't help to develop a healthy bond in the long
term. It **never** benefits a baby to have a rubber teat in its mouth and to
have its pleas ignored.

A dummy is **never** what a baby or child needs. I'll say that again because
it can not be overemphasised. **A dummy is NEVER what a baby or child
needs.** It's always a *replacement*, whether for food, love, or for comfort.

What are we avoiding by wanting our baby to 'shut up'? Is it their cry, or
our own discomfort, that we seek so desperately and quickly to quieten?
What are we closing off in *ourselves* that leads us to not only deny the
baby's need, but also ask it to accept an *artificial* and entirely inadequate
substitute for its mother's love and attention?

A mother's role is to see what it is her baby needs, and to help her child
achieve contentment. Dummies are always a sign that something is missing
in the mother-child relationship. We don't help anyone by pretending differently. My advice is, don't even start on a dummy. Be creative, be confident, be committed to mothering. Learn to recognise your baby's language.

A mother's nipples are self-cleaning. Dummies, on the other hand, har-
bour all sorts of nasty bugs, and need to be cleaned several times a day.
They also leach toxins into the baby's mouth.

Look around you, carefully. People are always putting something in their
mouths ~ food, fingers/thumbs, cigarettes, pens, hair. We have a cultural
compulsion to 'suck on something'. And how many of us, if we're honest,
do this when we're emotionally out of balance, even if only slightly? Usually
we aren't even conscious of such actions and habits.

By giving our child a dummy, or by not breastfeeding, we're setting
them up for a *lifetime* of sucking on something to deal with their emotional
pain. Food is often used, too, to cover our emotional pain, to numb our
feelings. More importantly, breastfeeding substitutes in childhood or adulthood *never* fill the need of not having been fully breastfed in childhood.

A mother is vital in showing her child, through her own example, how to
discover healthy ways of meeting needs.

The Drinks Are On Me

...en who have chosen not to breastfeed, offer their child ...ng'? They can't. Women who can't comfort feed often then ...mmies, which are really an extension of the concept of bottle-
...
...he reduction in oxygen to the brain, by the use of bottles or dummies, ...as been shown in studies to suppress deep breathing, leading to a lower emotional and intellectual quota[51].

Tandem nursing

I'm so grateful that I had Bethany to breastfeed during those three long, emotionally horrific days in NICU. The first time my girls breastfed together it just seemed so natural, so right. My tiny infant, and my young, growing child, nursed side by side for nourishment and nurturing. I'll cover the subject of tandem nursing, where two siblings of different ages breastfeed together, later on.

Breastfeeding 'unfriendly' policy

I felt huge frustration that the hospital staff were so determined to give Eliza formula by tube when my breasts were full, and as huge as watermelons. I expressed milk and watched over her night and day! When she did finally get to feed at my breast, she made up for lost time and put on 750 grams in three days!

My experience during this very difficult week ignited a passion in me that burns very strongly to this day: a passion to protect families from unnecessary intervention. I feel deep compassion for women and babies who don't have a breastfeeding experience, or have it cut short, and have their physical and emotional needs met artificially. This compassion comes *not* from judgement, but from a deep understanding and knowledge of the human body, and a sense of 'there but for the Grace of God go I'.

Had I not had the support, experiences, inspiration and determination, my journey could have been entirely different. And my daughters may have been raised in a completely different way.

All around the hospital were posters declaring it to be Breastfeeding Friendly. In our experience, and from what we observed and have heard from many other parents, nothing could have been further from the truth.

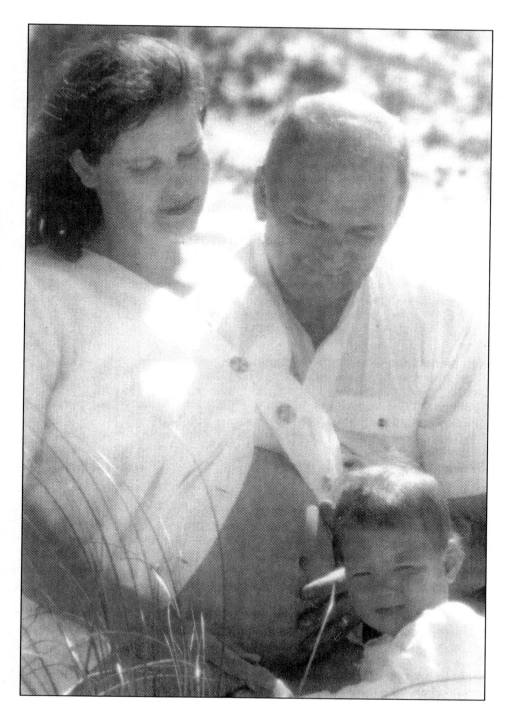

The Drinks Are On Me

Premature babies in NICU

My experience showed me an alarming situation which is played out in NICUs around the world. During our stay with Eliza, we rarely saw another mother tending to her premature baby. Each parent was told by staff, "there's nothing you can do, you may as well go home." This was confirmed over and over again when I asked staff where the parents were of these fragile, fit-in-your-palm babies. Even when premature babies are not capable of taking breast milk by mouth, they *need* to hear their mother, feel her skin, smell her. For breastfeeding to begin and progress well, the mother needs to remain with her premature baby as much as is humanly possible. She can feed her baby from a pipette or cup. The ideal way is to drip breast milk directly from the breast. Clearly, this is much easier if the parent is actively practising Kangaroo Care around the clock.

The best place for a premature baby to be is at home. Babies can be born at home from about 34 weeks as their lungs can work independently by this age. The priority is to ensure the baby receives kangaroo care. This involves keeping the baby warm, around the clock, by holding them inside your shirt against your chest. Babies raised this way do significantly better than premature babies kept in hospital[1].

Tips to welcome your premature baby home:
Make sure you have practical and emotional support. This is vital.
Become more involved with baby's routine while still in hospital.
Learn to breastfeed on cue while in hospital (that is, before baby cries) to develop the practice before you get home.
Keep baby close to you at all times/carry on your chest/maintain skin-to-skin contact.
Eat well and drink to thirst.
Rest.
Hire an electric pump ~ ideally a dual pump.
Learn signs of successful breastfeeding
Record changes in your baby - even if they seem small and insignificant. This may help you feel confident that your baby is growing and developing. There's a balance between trusting your intuition and keeping conscious of changes.
Avoid nipple confusion - don't use dummies, bottles, etc.

If you have a premature baby, you're likely to feel an overwhelming mixture of emotions, maybe even a sense of shock and grief; you may even be in denial that your baby has been born early and is having medical care. Don't be surprised if you feel guilt, anger, fear and confusion. This is common for the mother of a premature baby. You could also feel emotionally numb, depressed and experience a state of anxiety.

It's not uncommon for the parents of babies in special care to be bullied by staff and told 'there's nothing you can do'. This is *your* baby and you have every right to be there. **Your baby needs you.** Try and spend as much time with her as possible, and remember, there is plenty you can do. There are often guidelines drawn up by the hospital and even by La Leche League as to the minimum weight a baby should be before you can breastfeed and hold her. Always, *always*, draw on your own strength and what you feel is right for your baby.

You can begin kangaroo care (holding baby close) 24/7. Remember, this is the true meaning of kangaroo care, not the hospital definition of an hour a day.

If baby's apgar score at birth was 6 you can breastfeed immediately. Even one week of breastfeeding provides protection against infection. Is your baby needing to be fed through a tube? This is the time to be express-ing breast milk. **Every drop is vital.** Imagine each drop containing a life-time's worth of nature's immunisation. Try and hold baby, or touch him, before pumping. Put a breast pad with your milk near to baby in his crib, so that he can recognise your smell.

Donor milk, while infinitely better than formula, is pasteurised, which kills the live cells that fight infection. So try to use an automatic electric piston pump, and have your own milk available. A double pump takes half the time. **No amount of milk is too small.** *Every drop of your early milk is valuable, and unique to your baby.* When pumping, mimic the feeds of your baby. Pump ten to fifteen minutes on each breast every two hours. Keep a regular routine. The more you stimulate the breasts, the more milk you will make. It will trigger the milk-making hormones. The rhythm of a premature baby may be different to a baby born at term.

The expression of breast milk is an emotional and a physical skill. Expect to take time to learn how to do it. Don't give up because of impatience. Learn to relax, and then you'll achieve an effective let-down. Avoid having an audience.

The longer you pump, the more the fat content of your milk increases. Aim for at least 100 minutes a day. Touch your baby, to reduce your own anxiety. If pumping hurts, try a different pump. Don't be coerced into be-lieving formula is the best for a pre-term baby. The formula milk industry is a big business, and hospital staff are regularly approached by international companies to promote their products! Have a look at all the sponsored 'goodies' in the nurses' station.

Pre-term milk contains *even more* infection-fighting antibodies than that of term mothers. You see, Nature doesn't miss a trick. Your first few feeds with baby at breast will take a lot of time, patience and privacy. You'll need to be well supported with cushions. Aim to nurse well, from at least one breast.

The Drinks Are On Me

It will probably take several sessions for baby to get used to breastfeeding. The first goal is to get your babe interested in licking and recognising the nipple. Breastfeeding should not be delayed. Many studies show that it is less stressful than bottle-feeding[2].

Some helpful tips:
Touch and talk to your baby a lot.
Try and stay with your baby around the clock if possible, or set up a rota with family members and friends.
Change and feed your baby as much as possible.
Use your baby's name often. Tell her that you love her, and are glad she's in your life.
Ask questions of the staff.
Don't be afraid to offer suggestions.
Put photos of yourself and your family in the crib. If you can't be with baby, leave a tape recording of your voice.

Remember:
Breast milk is easier to digest (only takes 20 minutes) than formula.
The breastfeeding rhythm/pattern is established between mother and baby earlier than with formula feeding.
Antibodies protect against bacterial infection.
Breastfed babies have improved motor development.
Breastfed babies have higher intelligence and better vision. Let's put this into perspective though. Breastfed babies are **as nature intended,** not better. Bottle-fed babies are **compromised**[3].

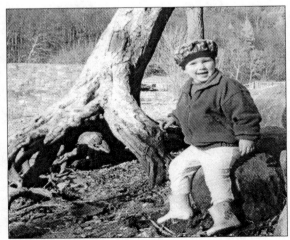

Eliza enjoying toddlerhood, her days and nights enhanced by a breastfeeding relationship.

The Drinks Are On Me

Engorgement, plugged milk ducts and mastitis

The state of overly full breasts, known as engorgement, tends to occur a few days after birth. It's recognised by a low-grade fever, which lasts 12 - 48 hours. Use warm, moist compresses. Frequently feed your baby. Make sure baby is well positioned and has a good latch-on. Try a gentle breast massage. Use the palm, and move it down towards the nipple. It's particularly effective in a warm shower. Normal fullness in breasts doesn't hurt, though it may be uncomfortable.

If you have a plugged duct, a tender spot or lump in the breast, keep breastfeeding. The duct became inflamed because milk wasn't able to flow freely. Is your bra too tight? Is baby latched-on properly? Positioned correctly? Has it been too long between feeds? Is there dried milk covering the nipple opening?

Rest.
Apply heat.
Nurse often. Take baby to bed and do nothing!
Change nursing positions regularly.
Ask for help with household duties. Your *only duty* at this moment is to be with your baby and rest. Don't stop breastfeeding.

Mastitis

Mastitis is inflammation of the breast. It can come from an untreated plugged duct. Some women experience fever and flu-like symptoms. It tends to occur when a breastfeeding mother is tired and run down. If it's still there after 24 hours, see a health-care professional.

Be sure to tell your health-care provider that:

Studies show it's best to keep feeding and not wean[52].
Antibodies in the milk protect the baby from bacteria.

If you opt for antibiotics, take all of the prescribed medication, to prevent mastitis recurring. Take a pro-biotic to refurnish healthy gut bacteria. Ensure you have a balanced diet. Limit your activities to just nursing.

Medications may reduce milk supply, as can breast injuries and operations. Both pregnancy and the oral contraceptive pill can inhibit milk supply, as can being a smoker, and having a retained placenta. Birth injuries, jaundice, a sick baby with a cold, ear and urinary tract infections may impact on milk flow.

The Drinks Are On Me

If your baby has green stools, try to keep him on the breast for longer. It could be a foremilk imbalance. Switch breasts during feeds to keep baby interested, and able to receive hindmilk. Offer both breasts at least twice, and nurse for at least thirty minutes. Switch sides when baby's sucking and swallowing slow down.

Plugged milk ducts
A plugged duct is a sign you're doing too much

The milk ducts sometimes get 'plugged'. This means you'll see and feel a tender area beneath the areola. You won't feel ill, as with mastitis, though you might experience pain on occasion. It does need tending to though, as it can lead to infections. It's important that you continue breastfeeding from the affected breast. The milk is not harmful to your baby. If you feel too sore to breastfeed, then express, or stand under a warm shower and use your palm to push milk down your breast towards the nipple. By starting your baby on the sore breast first, he'll have the most strength to help re-move the milk, and is unlikely to fall asleep on the job! As ever, ensure good latch-on so that all the milk can be drained.

Prevention is better than cure
If you consider your nipple to be like a watch, with different time posi-tions around the areola, you'll get an idea of the milk ducts all leading to the centre. Try different feeding positions, so the baby is effectively com-ing at the ducts from all angles, to drain the breast.

Poultice
I learnt about making a poultice from my mum. Years ago, she was acci-dentally shot in the chest by campers, when out for an afternoon stroll with my dad. The bullet lodged itself so close to the lung that the doctors could-n't operate without the risk of severely damaging the lungs. She made her-self a poultice from squashed grapes to 'draw out' the bullet.

If you've got engorged breasts or mastitis, you can use a holistic remedy for treating this discomfort. And if you've never experienced engorgement, you're a lucky girl. It makes you feel like you've got rocks on your chest, rather than soft, squidgy breasts. And then there's the fever...but enough of that. Here's what you need to know: obtain fenugreek seeds, and soak them in a cup of boiling water. Once they've cooled down, grind or mash them up. Put them in a warmed-up, clean towel or nappy, before placing on your breasts. It will allow them to let milk down again.

Slow or low weight gain is commonly a result of breastfeeding misman-agement, not to mention the very odd and pointless practice of using meas-urement charts from the 1970s, based on babies who were bottle-fed, and fed on a schedule. New charts are slowly being introduced to the UK, but they are still inadequate because they are not based on child-led breast-feeding practices.

Signs of inadequate intake in a newly breastfed baby
is listless
has a sunken fontanelle
is not waking to nurse at night
has fewer than ten feeds a day
has a dry mouth and/or eyes
has a weak cry
is lethargic

You can increase milk by
checking positioning and latch-on
nursing frequently
offering both breasts at each feed so baby gets hindmilk
avoiding bottles and pacifiers
eliminating formula
taking care of mother

Safe herbs for a mother to increase milk include fennel, fenugreek and caraway seeds. You can stew them into a tea, eat straight, or soak and sprout for use in salads.

Slow weight gain means the baby has a consistent weight gain and mile-stones are being met. He has soft stools, pale urine (6 wet nappies), is alert, sucks and swallows actively, feeds frequently and has good muscle tone. The mother experiences let-down. There is very little biological rea-son for not being able to breastfeed. Women who have difficulties, for any reason, should contact their nearest breastfeeding counsellor.

Failure to thrive
dehydrated
greyish
strong urine
still losing weight after ten days
inadequate stools
refusal to feed from birth
birth weight not regained after 3 weeks
weight loss greater than 10% of birth weight by 7-14 days

The Drinks Are On Me

loss of fat layer
malnutrition
lethargic
little or no growth in head circumference or body length
weight below ten percentile

Please see a health care provider (experienced with breastfeeding) or a La Leche League Leader, who understands your baby's breastfeeding needs. It's considered 'normal' for a baby to lose from 5 - 10 % of its birth weight. It's usually regained within two to three weeks. Gain should be determined on lowest weight (around four days old). At three to four months, a baby would be gaining about 113 - 227 grams per week (four to eight ounces). Birth weight doubles by about five to six months.
Length growth is usually 2.5 cm a month.
Head circumference increase is about 1.27cm a month.
Always remember though, that every baby is unique and has its own rate of growth.
Breast milk should be the sole source of food for __at least__ six months, though ideally nearer to eight or nine months.

Breastfeeding and AIDS

It's not known if babies acquire Human Immunodeficiency Virus (HIV) from their mother in utero, or through drinking breast milk. Studies show that the majority of babies who have mothers with HIV do not become infected through drinking breast milk[4&5]. Vitamin A deficiency in the pregnant mother has been linked to the foetus being infected with HIV. Both World Health Organisation and UNICEF (1992) recommend that breastfeeding should continue in children born to HIV mothers, because the risk of death from *other* causes is likely to be high if the child is not breastfed.

A Danish pasteurising device has provided breakthrough treatment for HIV-infected breastfeeding mothers. Pasteurising their infected breast milk at 60 degrees Celsius for 30 minutes, using solar power, inactivates HIV and pathogenic bacteria. This means a nursing mother is able to operate a pasteuriser herself for under $100 US a year. Anti-viral medication for HIV costs up to twelve thousand dollars per year. Dr Jorgensen, of Kolding Hospital in Denmark, says that the antibodies are unharmed during the milk pasteurisation process. Dr Jorgensen is a specialist in tropical and infectious diseases, and has worked for the National AIDS Control Programme in Tanzania. As to be expected, the pharmaceutical industry has not been supporting or promoting the pasteurising concept. This device is still new ground, and studies show it's safer and better for these babies to directly receive their mother's breast milk.

Caesareans and breastfeeding

A caesarian section is not to be undertaken lightly. It should never come under the category of a lifestyle choice. It should be reserved exclusively for medical emergencies. It would take a whole book to write why it's important for babies mentally, physically and spiritually to undergo the journey of being born out of their mother's birth canal.

Many women are unaware that this major abdominal surgery to remove their baby will impact on their ability to breastfeed. Those who are aware, often believe it's because of the surgery itself.

Although this is a factor, the biggest disruption to initiating successful breastfeeding is the injection of *morphine* into the mother, as a painkiller. Studies have shown it has a huge impact on the mother's oxytocin secretion, and *inhibits* her natural ability to make milk. It doesn't make it impossible by any means, but it's something all mothers should consider before going under the knife.

All the rules of supply and demand still apply to mums who have their baby delivered by caesarean. Don't give up! Create a safe haven for initiating breastfeeding. Drink plenty of water to detox the drugs from your system. Have a regular supply of nettle tea to aid elimination of morphine, and alternate with fennel tea to boost your milk supply.

Ask for your baby to be put straight on your chest after birth. There's no need for eye wipes, vitamin K injections, heel pricks, weighing and washing. The *only* thing your baby needs is you. You and your baby have the *right* to have immediate skin contact and to initiate breastfeeding.

Although you may feel fine, your baby has just undergone a major shock. In all cases she'll be compromised by the drugs she's received from you via the placenta. A caesarean-born baby does not arrive in optimal shape. Her body hasn't done things that she was *biologically* expecting to do in birthing. Delayed breastfeeding after surgery also compromises the baby.

From her warm, comfortable, dimly lit and safe little world ~ the only one she's known while being in a physical body ~ without warning, she's been pulled out into an alien environment of loud noises, harsh lights, rough hands, strangers and gravity. This is immensely shocking to any newborn baby. Hormones will be coursing through her veins as she tries to make sense of her new world; however, she will interpret them as fight or flight messages of death and fear, rather than love.

Be kind, be considerate, and put the baby's needs before anything else. If you're physically incapable of holding your baby, ensure your partner, mother or best friend, provides skin-to-skin contact.

The Drinks Are On Me

Gently talk to your baby. Explain what's happening. Allow your *love* hormones, the givers of life, to surge from you and into your baby.

Breastfeeding straight after birth is always important, and no doubt even more so after the rude shock of a caesarean delivery.

Be gentle with yourself. You've just had major abdominal surgery, so rest, and don't lift anything heavier than your baby. Ensure you have lots of pillows around so that your back is well supported and you're comfortable breastfeeding.

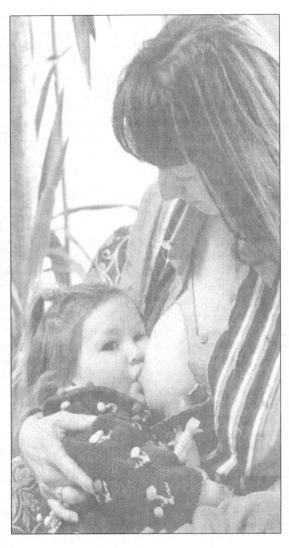

Cindy successfully breastfed her Daughter, Ginevee, full-term after a caesarean section.

Jaundice

Jaundice is a condition which causes yellowing of the skin, eyes and mucus membranes when bilirubin (a yellow-orange compound) is not removed from the body quickly enough by the liver. Early and frequent breastfeeding will prevent jaundice becoming exaggerated. A minimum of ten breastfeeding sessions are required per 24 hours. The first day is critical. Studies show that babies who nurse 7-11 times from birth receive 86% more milk on the 2nd day than babies who nurse fewer times[6]. Colostrum (the first rich milk) acts as a laxative. This is needed to pass meconium (bilirubin-rich first stools). When a jaundiced baby is feeding frequently and effectively, 'physiologic [normal] jaundice' will resolve on its own, without intervention. Jaundice is not a disease. It is harmless. It has no side-effects provided it doesn't reach unsafe levels. Interestingly, it's more prevalent in Chinese, Japanese, Korean, Native American and South Americans who live at higher altitudes. Lower oxygen levels lead to an increase in haemoglobin and red cells.

Don't be concerned if it takes two to three months to drop to adult levels. Some doctors recommend weaning, to determine if mother's milk is a factor. This is **not** beneficial, and is detrimental! Be aware that a high bilirubin count can increase sleepiness. You can always contact your local breastfeeding group, such as La Leche League, and ask for their medical team's research documents and studies.

Remember 10-12 feeds per 24 hours. That is, at least two-hourly, with one sleep of four to five hours. Some research indicates that higher bilirubin may be associated with *decreased* incidence of some diseases in term and preterm babies.

Try massaging your breasts to increase volume and fat content of milk.

Tips for the mother of a jaundiced baby
Undress baby and allow indirect sunlight onto its skin.
State that you don't want baby on supplements/dummy.
Insist that you want to spend time with your baby and have <u>uninterrupted</u> breastfeeding time.
If your baby needs bili lights, have them in your room.
Investigate phototherapy. Phototherapy babies are less likely to wean prematurely.
Suggest Wallaby phototherapy (fibre optic blanket).
Avoid aspirin (salicylates); sulfa drugs risk brain damage when baby is jaundiced[52, 55]. They shouldn't be used by a pregnant mother either[7].
Water supplements are to be avoided as they are associated with high bilirubin levels. Only 2% of bilirubin is eliminated through the urine. The bowels are the main evacuation point. Ninety-eight percent is eliminated through the bowels. Water will *not* stimulate bowels.

The Drinks Are On Me

Dehydration is not a contributing factor to jaundice, but low calories are! State to your doctor that studies show mothers of jaundiced babies are less likely to keep breastfeeding. Enlist his/her support in maintaining regular breastfeeding.

Breastfeeding should continue unless jaundice is found to be caused by a metabolic disease, such as galactosaemia. A doctor may be required to do tests to verify.

Tongue tie ~ short frenulum

My youngest brother, Albert, was born with a short frenulum, a condition otherwise known as tongue tie. My mum was unaware of this until he went to school and a dentist pointed it out to her. Tongue tie can affect speech development, but even more importantly, the ability to breastfeed successfully.

Tongue tie means that the frenulum, attaching the tongue to the floor of the mouth, is shorter than usual. Not all tongue tied babies experience difficulty with breastfeeding. It's also worth remembering that often a frenulum will loosen in time. To determine if your baby's frenulum is posing a problem, ask yourself the following, and if you're concerned seek specialist advice:

Is my baby happy breastfeeding?
Is latch-on painful?
Is my baby getting enough milk? (count wet nappies)
Does the tip of my baby's tongue come out past the bottom gum?
Does the tongue curl upward when my baby cries? If it curls under,
then it's too short.

Clipping the frenulum gives immediate results for breastfeeding. Latch-on is easy, effective, and mother and child are comfortable. Your doctor or midwife will be able to clip the frenulum quickly and easily. Apparently it's painless, but you can always ask for a local anaesthetic, and also ask for information about the ingredients it contains.

Cleft lip/palate

A baby with a cleft lip or palate is able to breastfeed. Unlike a rubber teat, the mother's nipple and breast are flexible and work with the baby's mouth. It's easier for the baby to adapt to the flow of milk from a breast, rather than a bottle. Breast milk is the optimal milk for a babe with a cleft lip or palate. Sometimes, if there's an opening in the palate, the milk can leak into the baby's nose. Although breastfeeding will be easier after surgery, initially it may be necessary to express milk for your baby in order to stimulate milk supply. You can feed this off your finger, in a pipette or a cup. If your doctor is unaware of either the benefits of breastfeeding, or that babies with a cleft lip/palate can breastfeed, then consult with a breastfeeding professional.

It's very common for babies with a cleft lip and palate to suffer from ear infections ~ one consequence of being raised on formula milk. You can avoid this by breastfeeding. As with other babies, correct latch-on is important so that the baby can effectively suckle all the milk. Creating a seal around the nipple can initially be challenging for babies with a cleft lip/palate.

Just remember, breast tissue is soft and flexible; this makes feeding these babies a lot easier than doing so with a bottle. I can't recommend highly enough seeking out the help and support of a competent lactation consultant, to guide you through the early days. She'll help you find breastfeeding positions which work best for your baby. Usually this is some sort of sitting position, to prevent milk going up your baby's nostril.

Breastfeeding multiples

Whether you breastfeed twins, triplets or more, it's important that you're fully supported, so that you can focus completely on being a mother.

Your breastfeeding experience will be enhanced by help from others around the house ~ meal preparation, household chores, playing with older children. It's important you get adequate rest, so sleep when your babies sleep! It may be possible to feed each of your babies one at a time; however, in the early days they may need to be fed simultaneously.

Tend to your nursing sanctuary ~ make it your haven, and fill it with lots of comfy cushions and pillows so that you're well-supported at each feeding session. Have someone ensure that any visitors are fully aware that you're *not* there to entertain. Let *them* make the cup of tea; and ask them to hang out the laundry while they wait for the kettle to boil.

It's so tempting for visitors to get all broody and stay over-time. Be clear with them that during these early days you need to conserve your energy for yourself and your babies. Your local breastfeeding counsellor or group leader will be able to guide you on various positions which work well for feeding two babies at once, or managing the feeding of more than two babies.

Down's Syndrome

It's a myth that babies with Down's Syndrome can't breastfeed. All babies need breast milk, and thrive on breastfeeding. As with other babies, correct information and support is important to a successful breastfeeding relationship. What makes a Down's baby different when it comes to breastfeeding is that they have lower muscle tone and have to be taught and encouraged to co-ordinate their sucking and swallowing with breathing. It's common for them to tire easily. Putting a Down's baby on a bottle in the hope of making it easier for them to feed is unhelpful.

The Drinks Are On Me

Breastfeeding helps them to develop their facial muscles. Clearly, the more they breastfeed, the easier it will become.

Don't compare your baby's growth to other babies, just look for all the usual signs that he's getting enough milk ~ such as wet nappies.

It's helpful to express a little milk onto your nipple at the start of breastfeeding so that he's able to taste milk sooner. Some women warm their breasts with a wet cloth or in a hot shower to facilitate let-down. As with all babies, ensure correct latch-on. Down's babies are known for having a poorer immunity than other children. Breastfeeding increases immunity, and the skin-to-skin contact is vital for health and well-being. Contact a lactation consultant or breastfeeding counsellor as soon as you're aware your baby has Down's, so that you can educate yourself on the best positioning and other helpful advice.

Vitamin D

Vitamin D is necessary for healthy bones and calcium absorption.

It would be wrong to conclude that breast milk is naturally low in vitamin D. The issue isn't about breast milk not being adequate for our children, but that the lactating mother isn't getting enough sunlight. We need to address the cause, not the symptom. Both mother and baby should be getting daily sunlight on their skins. It's very easy to do and shouldn't be avoided simply because we live in a sun-phobic culture.

There's an irony that vitamin D deficiency is being seen in sun-rich countries. Sunglasses, sunscreens and dark windows all prevent absorption of this necessary health ingredient. Our skin *makes* vitamin D when it's exposed to the sun's ultraviolet rays. When we wear sunglasses, our eyes are fooled into thinking there isn't much sunlight around, so they don't send a message to the skin, via the brain, to prepare for ultraviolet rays. Put simply, in order to know when your body has had enough sunlight, don't wear sunglasses.

By exposing your skin adequately in summer, your body is able to carry its stores into the winter months. Healthy sun absorption doesn't involve burning, it means introducing your skin gently and slowly to sunlight. Use early mornings and evenings to build up your tolerance levels gradually. Everybody needs sunlight.

Healthy bones and teeth are dependent on vitamin D. Deficiency has been connected to autoimmune diseases and osteoporosis later in life.

The main risk factor with skin cancer is not the sun, but our consumption of *unhealthy* oils. If your diet consists of fats found naturally, through raw seeds, nuts and leafy greens, rather than margarine, butter, fried foods, etc., your body will not be prone to skin cancer[8].

Nurturing the nurturer

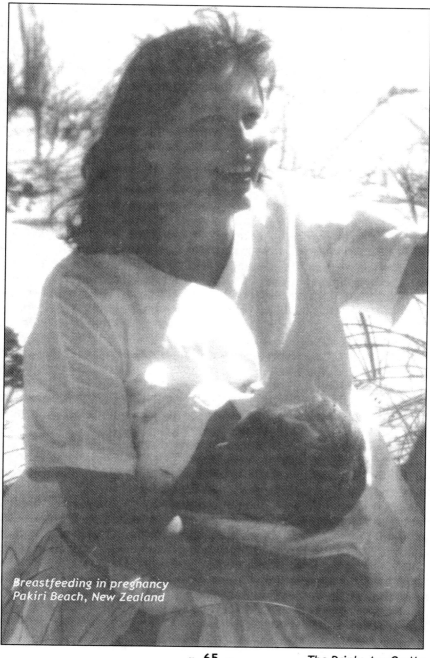

Breastfeeding in pregnancy
Pakiri Beach, New Zealand

The Drinks Are On Me

Drinking in our mother

When we breastfeed we take in our mother's emotional energy. As mothers, it's inevitable that we won't be bouncing along like Tigger all the time. Life throws us spanners sometimes. There may be grief, torment, frustration, despair, upset; all sorts of things can throw us off balance. It's important we continue to breastfeed, but we should remember than even if our child is non-verbal, we can *explain* what we're feeling and why we're feeling it. We can use our breastfeeding sessions to remind ourselves and our baby of the incredible love we share. It can glue us together even more in times of difficulty. My own mother recalls when her younger siblings died, her mother asked the remaining children to breastfeed, in order to relieve her full and aching breasts. My mother, to this day, remembers the feeling of drinking not only breast milk, but her mother's sorrow and grief.

Nursing station goodies

Creating a sanctuary, especially if new to breastfeeding, allows us to step into that space mentally, as well as physically. We draw our inner resources together and know that we're about to feed our baby consciously. Breastfeeding can happen anywhere, at any time, and with experience you'll perfect Breastfeeding Gymnastics. In our own home, though, it's helpful to know there's a special place. Even if you're breastfeeding on cue every twenty minutes, a sanctuary allows you to ritualise the experience. I've found it helpful to either have a bed, sofa or really comfy chair as the central piece of my sanctuary. Then I'd place on a nearby table a bowl of fresh fruit (easily accessible types, like grapes, are great). Dried fruit is wonderful if you've been busy and want a quick fix of energy. Don't rely on it though, as it's high in sugar. Water is a must, and should be the first drink of choice. If you really dislike the taste of water because you weren't brought up drinking it, then add a slice of fresh, organic lemon or fresh mint leaf. Avoid commercial lemon juice, it's full of e numbers and preservatives, and contains no enzymes. Warm water with fresh lemon is nice, too. If the water is warm, it eases digestion.

Your sanctuary can be a place of perfect peace, of absolute quiet, or you can have gentle, digestion-enhancing music like Mozart. Avoid music that disturbs the soul or creates a sense of needing to be active. Flute and watery music are great for letting down breast milk.

Some new mums keep a diary in their sanctuary. They record feeds and numbers of wet nappies, as well as how they're feeling, or the interactions they're having with their baby. Once your baby falls asleep at the breast, you might like to use this time for quiet reading. Keep a selection of inspirational reading material in your nursing sanctuary.

Looking after ourselves as mothers should be a priority, yet very sadly in our culture, we tend to end up at the back of the queue. Many women complain of being sore in the upper back. You can eliminate this by being conscious of your breastfeeding positions.

Keep your hips evenly apart, with a straight, well supported back. Good posture is vital. You can do simple Pilates or yoga positions to bring flexibility to your body. Women who enjoy regular cranio-sacral therapy or chiropractic care, find it helpful for staying in a state of ease.

I really enjoyed breastfeeding in the bath, as it meant my body was warm and relaxed, and my delicious baby got to wiggle her toes in the water.

A breastfeeding mother drinks a lot! Try to avoid commercial drinks, and stick to pure water and home-made juices. Your appetite will increase like nothing you've ever experienced. Don't deny the need to eat. Breastfeeding burns loads of calories. However, this isn't an excuse to gorge on cream buns. You're making breast milk 24/7. You are what you eat. And so is your baby. She is 100% reliant on your conscious healthy food choices from at least two years before conception, throughout pregnancy, and for the duration of breastfeeding, not to mention the example you set through her childhood[9].

NAK

There's no place for a tv or computer in your breastfeeding sanctuary. A modern phenomenon has swept the breastfeeding world, and this is of mums who NAK. Nursing At Keyboard is multi-tasking dysfunction. Babies need *conscious* mothers, and never more so than when they're at the breast. The world won't stop because you have to sit down and be with your baby while she feeds. I'm often alarmed at the number of women on e-groups who are sitting at computers with brand new babies on their laps, while they engage with cyber-mates. More often than not, the same mums also have toddlers who are *desperate* for their attention. Everyone misses out with NAK. The internet has opened up a whole new world, which enables mums to get invaluable information to help them with their parenting. We honour our babies best of all when we don't use *their* feeding time to access information or engage in cyber friendships.

It's important that babies develop rhythm when they learn to breastfeed, and a mum's job is to provide a calm and peaceful environment for baby to consume her meal.

Although on the one hand it's important that babies are part of our every day life and activities, you should always ask yourself if it's enhancing your breastfeeding relationship to have the baby so close to a machine which emits electromagnetic radiation.

If we're to parent holistically and consciously, full awareness and understanding of the impact of electromagnetic fields emitted from computers and televisions are necessary. It's one thing to subject ourselves to them, but do we have the right to inflict it on the very people who depend on us for their well-being?

Electro-stress impacts the neuro-chemical pathways to the pituitary and pineal glands, as well as the endocrine system. For babies, the best light is natural daylight.

The Drinks Are On Me

Being exposed to the fluorescent lighting of a computer or television can lead to hyperactivity, less resistance to disease, heart illness, aggressive behaviour, and cancer.

Sometimes the effects of radiation simply aren't visible to us, yet evidence from the US National Council of Radiation Protection shows long term effects on human health[10].

Journaling

Anyone can keep a journal, it's not just for people who consider themselves writers. Journaling allows us space to review and reflect. It acts as a witness to our journey.

The following questions are designed to help you explore your attitudes towards breastfeeding. You might like to use a special notepad to record your thoughts. If a question feels difficult, stick with it, because it will help you enormously to uncover your deeper beliefs. When we know our deeper driving forces, it helps us to be more tolerant of ourselves and other people.

Did your mother breastfeed? What was/is her attitude to breastfeeding?
Was your baby born at term?
When did your baby first go onto the breast?
Did your baby get colostrum? (The rich, thick milk that is produced in the first few days after birth).
Did baby latch well? Are baby's lips flanged, that is, spread well around the areola? (the pink area around the nipple).
Can you hear baby swallowing?
Does baby have 6-8 wet nappies a day?
How do you feel about breastfeeding in front of other people?
What do you consider to be the benefits of breastfeeding for mother and baby?
What are some things you can do to make breastfeeding a time of pleasure and comfort?
Consider breastfeeding from your baby's point of view. How are you satisfying your baby's needs?
Do you feel supported by your partner?
What suggestions could you offer to increase your partner's support for you?

Journaling questions for dad:
How do you feel about breastfeeding in general?
How do you feel about your partner breastfeeding?
What feelings do you have when you see your baby suckling from your part-
ner?
Do you think women should be able to breastfeed in public? Why? Why not?
Would you feel comfortable if your partner breastfed in front of your male
friends?
How long do you think a baby should breastfeed for?
Do you know the main reason women cease breastfeeding is because their
partner doesn't support them, or feels embarrassed[59]? What is your reac-
tion to this?
How can you support your partner and baby in their breastfeeding relation-
ship?

Here are some simple and effective ways to nurture yourself, as a mother, and especially as a breastfeeding mother:

Living foods
A living food is one where the enzymes in the food are still living. Why is it important that we eat living foods? The enzymes simplify the job of our digestive system, and are vital for vibrant health. Living foods include raw fruit, raw vegetables, seeds, nuts, fungi and sea vegetables. As soon as we heat foods to about 40 degrees Celsius, the enzymes are rendered useless. This doesn't mean that all nutrition is destroyed, though it is *severely* com-promised. Try having an 'all raw' meal, and see how differently you feel af-terwards compared to a meal of bread or baked potato, for example.

Incorporating more living foods in your meals will make a huge differ-ence both to your energy levels and breast milk production. Raw fruit and vegetables have a high water content, which is vital for our bodies, given that we, too, are mostly made of water. Many of us go through life never knowing how different we can feel by making different food choices.

Homeopathy
Many women have successfully used homeopathy to help treat various issues which come up in breastfeeding, such as mastitis and sore nipples. There are many self-help homeopathy books on the market; however, it is rather an exact science, so for something serious like breastfeeding issues, it's well worth consulting a homeopath.

The Drinks Are On Me

Cranio-sacral therapy and chiropractic care

When we become a parent, the joy can very quickly be replaced with upset and anguish if our little treasure cries non-stop. There are many reasons for unhappy babies. Many babies experience discomfort in the neck area from birth, especially if they've had medically managed births. Utilising cranio-sacral therapy or chiropractic care can make a big difference. It's important for mothers to emerge post partum intact, and happy too, so regular visits after birth should be a must. In some countries, for example, New Zealand, there are therapists who provide free sessions for babies for the first six weeks after birth. Take advantage of this generosity, because it really will make all the difference. These therapies are incredibly helpful during times of colic, teething and when there has been too much time spent in baby car seats.

Holistic support comes in many ways. Each of us has a preference for what nurtures us. You might like to explore and experiment with acupuncture, reiki, shiatsu, Bowen technique, colour therapy and chakra balancing.

Visualisation

Our imagination is more powerful than our will power. You can visualise your milk flowing abundantly, and you can also visualise being well-rested, nurtured, loved and loving. It's as simple as closing your eyes, and drawing the pictures in your mind as vividly as possible. The key to visualising is not just to make it a visual experience, but a 'felt' one, too. What does it *feel* like to really nurture your babies and children? What does it *feel* like to live in a happy home? What does it *feel* like to have a supportive partner or friends helping *you* to be a great mother? Allow yourself to live within the *feeling*, and soon it will be part of your everyday life.

Meditation

It's not uncommon for people who regularly meditate to suddenly give up the practice when they have a baby, because they believe there isn't any time. At one level this is true, because being a parent can be all-consuming. However, if, as parents, we deliberately create pockets of time to nurture our inner-self, we emerge more clearly and are able to be a better parent.

Meditation isn't just for bearded gurus in dark caves a thousand miles from civilisation. It's for everyone, and with a little practice, it's a simple and effective way of not only getting through stressful times, but of discovering our more intuitive selves. Being in touch with who we really are, rather than the self we show to others, enables us to move powerfully through our world, bringing health and happiness not only to ourselves and family, but to the world at large. And all this from a few minutes of quiet each day? Yes indeed! There's no point setting a goal to meditate for half an hour if you've never sat still for more than five minutes in your life. Start with three minutes and then build up to five, ten and twenty. Make it easy and accessible for yourself.

Some people need silence for meditation, others need music. If you do use music, try something with an unpredictable melody, like many of the New Age compositions. You don't want music where your brain is going to follow the tune. Personally, I love to meditate after I've lit incense and a beeswax candle. I like the lights dimmed and gentle music. The key to meditation is to calm the mind. In doing so, the body is calmed. When our whole being is in this state, we're able to act more authentically. From here we start living our truth: from our truth, comes happiness.

I can't emphasise enough the difference a little time out will make to your day. Keep it short, keep it simple. It's a rare baby who won't sleep long enough to give you five minutes of peace. However, some little babies seem to be awake **all** the time. Bless 'em! It's helpful to remember that babies are constantly changing, and at some point your baby <u>will</u> sleep for extended periods.

Everything in mothering has the potential to be a meditation if we bring mindful awareness to the task at hand. Whether it's washing the dishes or changing a nappy, if we're in the present moment and fully connected in mind and body, then we're in a meditative state. It has been said that having a child is like having a live-in Zen Master. Raising children is an eighteen year meditation retreat! If you look at parenting in a positive light, and see it as a practice or path of lifelong meditation, it will help you celebrate each day.

Breastfeeding as meditation

Many women feel that breastfeeding is a demanding, 24 hour a day job. They're right. And many women feel they just don't have time for that commitment. My mother once told me that the best way to avoid responsibility is to accept it. This sounds like a contradiction, but what she meant was that when we *accept* a situation, melt into it, become part of it, then it loses its ability to overwhelm us. We no longer feel threatened or out of control.

It's not uncommon for women in our culture to feel resentment during their mothering. Sometimes they feel that way about breastfeeding, and believe weaning their child will bring an end to those feelings. The truth is though, the resentment goes much deeper than that, and we take those issues into other aspects of our parenting or marital partnership. The most helpful thing we can do when we find ourselves in that situation is to **own** the resentment. Acknowledging how we feel, and accepting that it's our own self which needs changing, rather than the child, empowers both mother and child.

Society, caught up in its fast-paced and instant gratification mode, doesn't encourage the birthright of every baby. Nature hasn't planned for this change of attitude. The price we pay for ignoring our biological expectations is very high.

Our babies are genetically *programmed* to expect to receive mother's milk around the clock. Their tiny bodies *expect* to have the nurturing arms of mother around them all the time. The reason that human milk is thinner than the milk of other mammals is because Nature designed it that our babies drink regularly and often. This is vital for the optimal brain development of higher species of animals. Nature doesn't want us separated from our babies, or for them to grow into cows!

We can come into mothering by recognising it as an essential part of our unique life purpose and to reclaim motherhood as sacred ground. No longer is it acceptable to drop our head and say "I'm just a mother". Stand tall, as there is no higher path to walk on this Earth than to birth babies, nurture at the breast, and to provide a living example of what it means to be a human and live with love. There's no greater reason to hold our head high than that of being a mother. Be proud.

If you've stepped out of the competitive commercial sector and landed head first into mothering, it can be like having a ton of concrete dropped on top of you. The journey becomes easier when you surrender and melt into mothering, rather than trying to avoid it by using things to keep you from your path.

Some women use daily affirmations to remind them of good mothering. Others will consciously go into their night dreams asking for guidance, visions and support as they navigate the parenting years. Ceremony is also a helpful way of honouring the rite of passage from maiden to mother. We have ceremonies for babies ~ namings, baptisms, placenta plantings, but how often, perhaps apart from a Blessingway, do we stop and honour motherhood? A ceremony after the birth of the baby, especially for the mother, where she is affirmed, could make all the difference in how a woman sees this part of her life. Our culture constantly undermines mothering, so whatever we can do to support ourselves and other mothers can only be a good thing.

The reason that human milk is thinner than the milk of other mammals is because Nature designed it that our babies drink regularly and often.

The Nips!

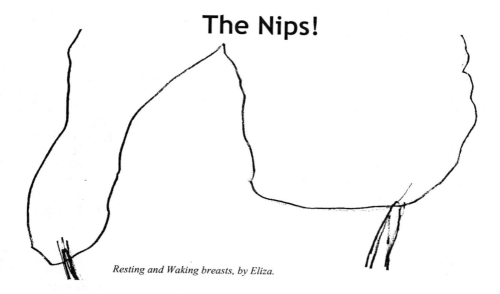

Resting and Waking breasts, by Eliza.

My daughter Eliza loved to call my nipples The Nips. Actually, she still affectionately refers to The Nips. Our nipples are one of the main tools in breastfeeding, so it pays to look after them. One of the most common reasons for stopping breastfeeding is cracked nipples. This is unfortunate, as it can be *easily* avoided with a little education. Cracked nipples are almost always caused from incorrect latch (that's right, blame the kid!). Another reason is if your nipples are always wet (soggy bra or breast pad). They need fresh air. One really useful tip, for sore nips, is to get two plastic tea strainers and cut the handles off. Sit one over each nipple, inside your bra. This will allow air to circulate, and any cracks to heal. It's probably best to remove the tea leaves first!

It's an instinctive reflex for a newborn baby to open her mouth when something touches her lip. This means she'll quite happily suck at a tiny part of your nipple unless you show and teach her otherwise. Show your baby how to latch-on properly, taking in the whole nipple and part of the areola. Learning this right at the start of breastfeeding will help to avoid the possibility of cracked nipples.

Twiddling

Once babies grow a bit, there comes a time when their hands start exploring mum's body during breastfeeding. This is cute when it first happens. Tiny fingers tugging on buttons, ear-rings and clothing. And then, *then* they discover the other nipple. This is *not* good. It should be *nipped* in the bud from day one. Oh, maybe the first time it's sweet, but then it becomes downright annoying, if not painful.

The Drinks Are On Me

Little ones soon become demonic in their determination to Twiddle the Nipple. Like biting, this is something that has to be stopped if you don't like it. Everyone handles Junior Twiddlers differently. Some mothers don't mind it at all.

Bringing an end to twiddling represents a first step in creating healthy boundaries. Our whole universe is made along laws and rules. Part of a healthy relationship is to say what we do accept and what we don't. It doesn't mean we don't love or care for the other, it means we love and care for ourselves too, and we're not doormats. I recommend, as much as possible, not having the other nipple on show or easily accessible to little chubby fingers. Instead, wear a necklace or something else you don't mind them fiddling with during feed time.

Some anthropologists have suggested that the nearest species to us also 'twiddle', and it is their way of creating and keeping 'attachment' between mother and child.

Nipple confusion

The difference between the way a baby extracts milk from your breast, compared to milk from a bottle, is huge. In order to avoid nipple confusion, don't give your baby a bottle unless in an emergency situation. A baby simply can't latch-on to a bottle teat in the same way she does on the breast. She can get confused and frustrated, and in many cases, the baby ends up refusing the breast and going for the 'easy' option of bottle-feeding.

Milk extraction from the breast requires a unique sucking motion not needed with bottle-feeding. On the breast, she has to open her mouth wide and draw the nipple and some of the areola right into the back of the mouth. Mothers should be wary of bottles deemed to be 'just like a breast'. Watch out for this insidious advertising, which seeks to undermine the uniqueness of breastfeeding.

To get milk from the breast, baby must coordinate tongue and jaw movements in a sucking motion that's unique to breastfeeding. Her tongue holds your breast against the roof of her mouth. Her gums draw on the bottom area of the areola, and the tongue draws the milk down into the nipple. A baby simply doesn't have to do this 'work' if she drinks from a bottle, as gravity allows it to 'fall' out. None of the oral and facial muscles which breastfeeding helps develop are necessary for bottle-feeding, and therefore won't have the opportunity to develop optimally. Nature, however, designed it for a baby to work for her milk, so she can develop strong jaw and face muscles. If your baby plays with a bottle, using habits such as sucking with the lips or gums, it will hurt your nipples if she tries the same thing. She'll also not suck enough milk from the breast, and end up diminishing the supply. Bottle-feeding gives the baby immediate milk, whereas to get the fore and hindmilk flowing, the baby needs to suckle for a minute.

Despite it appearing that bottle-feeding might seem like a breeze, studies show it is *far less stressful* for the baby to be breastfed, because her heart rate and breathing stabilise at mother's breast.

Less of her energy is actually required to breastfeed than bottle-feed[11]. Your baby can control the milk flow with her unique tongue action, swallowing and stopping when necessary.

If an emergency situation requires that you can't feed at the breast, rather than supplementing with a bottle, consider using a cup, teaspoon or pipette. It's infinitely better to avoid situations which lead to nipple confusion than to have to remedy it later. Dummies also lead to nipple confusion.

Before you have your baby, network with other women, ideally through breastfeeding groups; and make arrangements to wet nurse. I felt a lot more comfortable becoming a mum knowing there were women who felt as passionately about breastfeeding as me, and were happy to feed my baby from their breast in an emergency. Let's make wet nursing ~ for love, not money ~ a viable and sensible option again.

Re-educating your baby to feed at the breast after nipple confusion:
Get rid of all artificial nipple substitutes, including dummies.
Make breastfeeding a wonderful, sensual experience for your baby, with lots of eye contact, laughter, cuddles and skin-to-skin touch.
Breastfeed on cue ~ don't wait till the baby is distressed.
Remember all you learnt about breastfeeding: latching-on, positioning and ensuring baby's mouth is well open. If you can express a bit of milk before breastfeeding, she'll taste the milk immediately and feel inclined to keep sucking. Be patient. Be loving.

When we initiate breastfeeding with our baby, nerve pathways are created in her brain. This is her body's way of making the experience familiar, so that she knows what to do each time she breastfeeds. And with each feeding session the pathways become stronger. If you were to drive a car along the motorway every day and then were told to drive an aeroplane along a runway you'd be challenged, confused and probably a thousand other things besides! Yet this is what we expect of our babies when offering them a fake nipple.

Wet wound healing

Coastal women in Scandinavia often use small sea shells over their cracked or sore nipples. The enclosed space provides a micro-climate, which allows the wound to be surrounded by natural moisture, namely breast milk, which contains beneficial healing properties. This type of approach means the sores will not develop scabs, which dry off and bleed. You can try this yourself if you've got shells that cover your nipples without touching them. Some shells have sharper edges, so you may need to sand them down a bit.

The Drinks Are On Me

Preparing nipples for breastfeeding

When I was pregnant, someone advised me to scrub my nipples every day in preparation for breastfeeding. Wha*aaaaa*t? How insane. Why do women pass on such stupid information? It's not normal or natural for breastfeeding to hurt. There is very little reason why breastfeeding might hurt, and it's almost always because your baby isn't latched-on properly, or you've just lain down naked, boobs first, in a bunch of stinging nettles... or developed thrush or impetigo.

Have you noticed we don't call it nipple feeding, but breastfeeding? That's because when the baby is feeding properly, it takes in the areola as well as the nipple. It's really helpful to watch women who successfully breastfeed before you have a baby, so you can see what successful breast-feeding looks like. This is so much better than an illustration or photo in a book, simply because a breastfeeding baby's mouth isn't static.

Thrush

Thrush is a yeast infection which can give the mother tender, itchy nipples that are pink and flaky, and give the baby white spots inside its cheeks. Baby will usually have a nappy rash, and mum may have vaginal itching. Baby may make a clicking sound at the breast, and be fussy and gassy. It can take several weeks to get better.

Thrush *loves* a warm, dark and moist environment, such as mouths and vaginas. You can find this nasty little yeast infection, growing quick as jungle weed and having the time of its life, inside nappy-covered areas, flabby skin, and on nipples wet from soaked bra pads.

Signs of thrush include soreness, burning, itching, redness, blisters, shooting pains in your breast (during or just after a feed), and more often than not, when remedies for sore nipples aren't working! Tell-tale signs also include a baby having white, cottage cheese-like patches on the tongue and side of the mouth, and/or a yeasty nappy rash. Sudden soreness of nipples is your first indication of thrush, which is commonly brought about by antibiotics disturbing the intestinal flora of the gut.

Oral contraception can make a woman more inclined to get thrush. Other contributing factors include: antibiotics; having diabetes; living in a warm/humid climate; nutritional deficiencies such as vitamins A, B, C and K, iron & folic acid; steroids; dairy foods; sweet foods; and products high in yeast, such as bread, pizza and jam. Wet nursing pads should be replaced regularly.

thrush
hates
sunlight

Preventative measures for thrush
Always wash hands thoroughly
Nurse on the least sore side
Give baby short, frequent feeds
Break suction gently, inserting your little finger into the corner of baby's mouth and loosening her grip on the breast
Wash cloth pads in tea tree oil after each feed
Dry cotton pads in sunlight
Wash baby's sucking toys frequently
Let your nipples have as much access to fresh air as possible
Avoid commercial disposable breast pads, and make your own from cotton or hemp
Avoid bras made from synthetics

Tea tree oil is available for mother and baby, and is the best anti-viral and anti-bacterial product you can use. Apply it to your nipples (wash off thoroughly before breastfeeding, as tea tree is very strong), and also use in your washing.

Thrush hates sunlight, so give your nips a good suntan (don't burn them though!).

Nipple creams and ointments

The best care for your nipples is to rub them with your very own breast milk. It's rich in vitamin E, and is anti-bacterial. This practice should be avoided, though, if you think you may have a yeast infection, as yeast thrives in milk. Thrush is a symptom of our modern dietary habits. **Avoid** all processed sugars, and yeast. Eliminate bread too, and your thrush will clear up quickly. Commonly, Nystatin is prescribed for nipples infected by yeast. However, I don't recommend this, as yeast has become resistant to Nystatin, *and* because it's a band-aid solution to a <u>systemic</u> issue. Instead, attend to your diet.

Avoid any nipple cream with ingredients that are toxic to your baby, which essentially is anything mass-produced or given out in hospitals.

DIY natural nipple creams
Make your own natural nipple cream and then you can be sure the ingredients are safe. The following suggestions are helpful for all the usual nipple complaints:

Use paw paw cream, or ideally, fresh paw paw mashed into a puree. Then put it directly onto the nipple/s. Paw paw has even been known to clear up Golden Staph infections.
Mix raw apricot oil, calendula, lavender, grapeseed and chamomile oils. Apply directly to nipples.

The Drinks Are On Me

An effective and natural nipple cream can be made by blending a table-spoon of Shea butter (from the Shea tree) with a tablespoon of New Zea-land Manuka honey, available from good health food stores. (It must be high grade Manuka as it has rare healing properties). Combine with two drops of essential rose oil. Apply gently to nipples. The products are not toxic to mother and baby.
Some mothers have blended neem powder with Manuka honey and a drop of water for another excellent, natural nipple cream.

Lansinoh TM is a nipple cream often recommended for cracked nipples. Please be aware that it contains lanolin, a derivative of the sheep industry. You may not want to use a product which can only be obtained through harming another living creature.

Inverted nipples
If you've got flat or inverted nipples, you may not actually be aware of it until you come to breastfeed for the first time. It can initially make breast-feeding a more sensitive experience. You can learn to massage your nipple until it comes out. When it does so, using your index finger and thumb, roll the nipple for a couple of minutes. You're *educating* your nipple to stand erect. If you feel unsure, get lactation support, as inverted nipples are <u>not</u> a reason to bottle-feed. Research indicates that whether or not a mother 'works' the nipples to make them stand proud, she can breastfeed effec-tively. If you and your baby are comfortable, and he's extracting enough milk, then that's all that matters.

Impetigo
If you're unfortunate enough to experience impetigo, (caused by bacte-ria), resulting in open sores on your nipples, first, get some echinacea tea (or capsules) to build up your immunity. Tea would be better. Try and have raw garlic in your diet (or rubbed on the soles of your feet!), to help detox-ify.
For the nipples, use calendula lotion to soothe and disinfect. The best natural disinfectant, and the ultimate antifungal and antibacterial thing from nature you can use, is undiluted tea tree oil. Just dab it onto the in-fected area, neat. If it causes too much discomfort, i.e. stings, you may just have to use calendula, or lavender essential oil. Tea tree would work the quickest though.
Goldenseal speeds up healing, and dries up the wound. All these products are available in health stores. Garlic should be in your kitchen.
The most effective remedy for any sore nipple is fresh paw paw. As mentioned, this tropical fruit will clear up Golden Staph and impetigo. Sim-ply mash a little of the ripe fruit, and apply it to your nipples. Avoid wear-ing a bra, and let your skin get as much air as possible. Keep your nipple dry. And remember, if the door bell rings, don't answer the door topless.

Nipple pain

For some women, nipple pain can become excruciating. Like labour and birth, however, it's easy to set up a vicious cycle of fear = pain + more fear + more pain ~ simply because we're <u>expecting</u> it. By using our amazing abilities as a mother, to ride through difficulties, we may discover we have the skills to work through other challenging life circumstances.

Using simple breathing techniques, you can work through the nipple pain, and overcome discomfort. The tension a mother feels often diminishes once the milk has let down. She can choose to work through a challenge, rather than walk away from it, especially if she bears in mind that the situation is temporary. Learning how to relax is vital. When a woman is in a difficult situation, it's easy not to see the wood for the trees, and to confuse a temporary situation with a permanent one ~ thereby leading to the end of the breastfeeding relationship.

Deepak Chopra describes breathing as *"the junction point between mind, body and soul. Every change of mental state is reflected in the breath and then in the body."*

Although breathing is, for the most part, unconscious, it's actually under our conscious control, and we can use it to influence our bodily responses to pain. By not choosing to consciously use slow and deep breathing during difficult breastfeeding times, we set ourselves up for a fight or flight response, with the adrenalin essentially overriding the calming effects of our breastfeeding hormones. Adrenalin is like a 'death-rush' coursing through the body. Fear is contagious. As in birth, when someone around us is in a state of fear, it is passed on energetically. If the mother who is breastfeeding is feeling fear because she is expecting pain, then likewise, those around her ~ child, partner, family, doctor, will pick up on this energy.

Re-lactation after nipple problems

In some cases, women choose not to nurse through nipple pain when it affects both breasts. It's helpful to know that breast milk stays in the breast for three to five years after breastfeeding, so if a cessation has occurred, there's no reason for a woman not to consider re-lactation, assuming she wants to breastfeed her child. A toddler or young child won't lose their sucking reflex in the relatively brief time of the nipple pain. If they were weaned off the breast abruptly, they may not feel emotionally secure enough to come back to it initially, and may take some encouraging. You could try offering some expressed milk on a spoon or in a cup, or you could squeeze some milk from your breast, letting it drip from the nipple to encourage your child to taste it, and become reacquainted with the breast. As with any aspect of breastfeeding, if there's a will, there's a way ~ and usually a very dedicated mother!

Teething and colic

Teething is one of the first milestones we go through with our children. It's here our babies learn about discomfort, pain and how to deal with something unpleasant within their being. Some children get through teething a lot more easily than others. Sometimes we don't realise our children are teething until a few days later, when we suddenly make the connection that we've not been able to do 'anything' around the house for days on end.

I can't help but wonder if babies who've had unmedicated births cope better than those who've started life on drugs. Nobody wants to see their baby in pain, but it's really important not to automatically go for pain-killers. This sets our children up for never dealing with discomfort and pain, but seeking to dull it. This, in turn, then sets up a pattern for dealing with all discomfort, be it physical, emotional or mental, by numbing out.

My suggestions for teething include taking a warm bath with your baby. Don't use plastic baby baths, get into the habit of bathing together. You can use this as the ultimate relaxant in the day for both of you. Breastfeeding in the bath is easy and relaxing. Just make sure you're fully prepared before getting in. Have towels, clothes and heating ready. I liked to make a pot of chamomile tea and sprinkle drops of lavender essential oil into the bath. Although this is plenty to create a calm, relaxed atmosphere, you could play some soothing music during bath time, or better still, sing to your baby.

From mid-afternoon, avoid the tv, radio and computer. Keep electrical impulses to an absolute minimum. Use lanterns and beeswax candles for low-level, natural lighting. Avoid stimulants, such as coffee, tea, chocolate, coke and sugar. Enjoy simple foods, such as vegetables and legumes.

After the bath, give baby a massage with cold-pressed almond or sesame oil (not toasted), warmed in your hands. Make sure the room is warm. The ultimate natural analgaesic for your baby is breastfeeding. It really does provide comfort. You can also offer her a frozen celery stick to chew on.

This might seem like a lot of work, which completely goes against the grain of a fast-paced society, but I can promise you that it's worth putting time and love, rather than drugs, into your baby. It keeps the whole family calm and happy. The above guide for teething is also helpful for avoiding colic! The key with colic is to recognise that the baby is energetically tuning into her mother and picking up 'end of day' stress. To beat colic the easiest remedy is to do nothing! Use the mornings to prepare your evening meal and do other chores, so that from lunch time onwards you are simply being with your baby. Avoid visitors, errands or anything else which will take you away from being present.

Amber teething necklaces

An ancient and holistic remedy for teething pain is the use of amber necklaces. Now becoming quite common in western society, the baby wears one around its neck.

Amber comes from the fossil resin of extinct conifer trees, up to 90 million years old. The amber has many other uses, including the treatment of headaches, migraines, asthma, epilepsy, rheumatism, and calming the nerves. The amber works when rubbed against the skin. It creates an electrostatic charge, which benefits the nervous system. I didn't know about amber teething necklaces when my girls were little, but one daughter now wears one to help her with car headaches.

Freezing breast milk

It's very common these days for mums to express breast milk for feeding at a later time, usually by another person. Breast milk is created in age and stage specific ways, and by its nature, is meant to be fed when and as needed. Breast milk was not designed to see the light of day. It was always intended, and still is, to go direct from source, sterile and warm, into the baby's throat. The milk made by your body this morning is different to the milk that will be made tonight. And next week it will be different again. Unless we're talking life-saving reasons, breast milk should be given as it is made. Some women keep their milk in the freezer for months on end. However, if you're giving your 6 month old baby milk that you made when he was two months old, he won't be receiving the immunities necessary for his six month old body.

If you do choose to freeze your milk, don't defrost it in a microwave. Allow it to do so at room temperature, and *then* warm the bottle in a pot of hot water. Breast milk can look rather odd when you defrost it, as it starts to separate. Don't throw it out, and <u>don't compare it to milk from animals</u>. Human milk is thinner, and has a blue-ish tinge to it. This is normal.

Breastfeeding is free, and allows the mother flexibility to feed her baby at any time, anywhere. It's always sterile, at the right temperature and right on tap. The drinks literally are on you. There's no need for any equipment or preparation time, no need to clean up, and it helps you to remember to slow down and be present with your baby.

Light is destructive, and air contaminates breast milk, so think twice if you need to express milk. Breast milk from the breast is nature's choice.

Medications and breastfeeding

Women often stop breastfeeding when issued with medication. This is usually unnecessary. Don't rely on your doctor to know if a drug is breastfeeding-compatible! Thomas Hale's book, *Medications and Mothers' Milk* is available through http://www.ibreastfeeding.com. It is updated regularly and should be in every office of every health care professional involved with breastfeeding women.

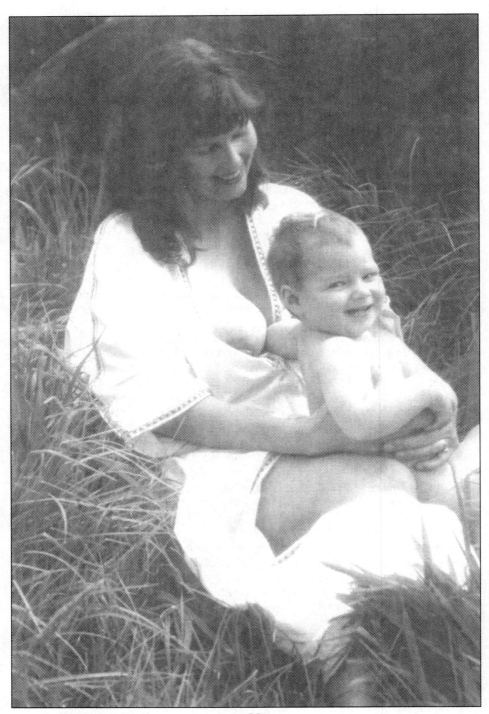

Isn't it poisonous?
Breastfeeding in pregnancy

Paul, Bethany and I were in a town hall, attending a psychic evening, when one of the mediums pointed me out and said another baby was coming along. 'No chance', I thought, 'I'm breastfeeding on cue'. Natural fertility and all that, I thought smugly. Idj*eeeee*t! Breastfeeding is a great natural contraception when you *exclusively* breastfeed.

If there's more than a six hour gap between breastfeeds, and your menstrual cycle or some bleeding has returned, then breastfeeding is **not** a 100% effective contraceptive. Interestingly, in a lot of cultures where the claim for breastfeeding as a contraceptive is derived, couples tend not to have sex in the first two years after their baby's birth. This paints a rather different picture to 'exclusive' breastfeeding being a natural contraceptive. These cultures hold the breastfeeding relationship sacred, and abstain from sex. Interestingly, tandem nursing in indigenous cultures is also rare, because abstinence naturally leads to a greater age gap between children. Most modern western women tend to have sex soon after giving birth, don't feed on cue, and are well nourished - so they can easily become pregnant again, as well as nurse through pregnancy and sustain two or more children at the breast.

Bethany had been eating a few different fruits, so was no longer exclusively breastfed at 15 months. I had one menstrual cycle, then 'bingo'.

It was once Eliza had made herself known, that a friend urged me to contact La Leche League, the international breastfeeding support group, promising me I'd find like-minded people there. I thought I'd give it a go. It was life-changing in so many ways.

I soon learnt there was no need to wean Bethany, and as long as we were both happy to continue the breastfeeding relationship, she could suckle right through pregnancy.

Funny what you learn from other people along the way though. "Isn't it poisonous for her to receive your breast milk when you're pregnant?" was just one of the many questions I fielded. Where on earth would anyone get an idea like that?

Bethany suckled away throughout my pregnancy. Near the end of gestation, however, my milk dried up, and I found her suckling excruciating. She didn't seem at all bothered by the lack of milk, though of course it's possible that she was extracting something, and I just didn't have the same ability when squeezing it out myself. Paul was invaluable at keeping her amused so I could get plenty of rest and relaxation.

The drying up of milk in pregnancy is very common. So common, that many toddlers use this time to self-wean. Not my Bethany; perhaps she knew what liquid gold was in store for her.

I believe the number one reason for a child weaning during the first few years of life, or in pregnancy, is because she *energetically* picks up her mother's discomfort and resentment at sustained breastfeeding. There's a lot of pressure on the child, from other people, to wean. In a place 'beyond' words, the child is hearing that breastfeeding is no longer acceptable.

One of my favourite images is of Bethany breastfeeding while I laboured in the birthing pool. It looked like we were both having a bit of fun in the spa! Bethany was 22 months old. In retrospect, she was such a little girl, and it must have really knocked her world upside down to have a baby come along then. Bethany's toddlerhood benefited enormously from the continuation of our breastfeeding relationship.

Eliza's birth was not the idyllic waterbirth at home that we'd planned. Instead, I was told it was 'illegal' to have a home-birth in NZ if you're more than ten days past your due date. Ironically, it wasn't until Eliza's fourth birthday that I found out that this is untrue, and a midwife's own policy can be over-ridden. Any policy can be overridden by a parent signing a disclaimer - taking responsibility, in writing, and accepting the outcome. Take back your power and do what you feel is right, rather than what you're told you 'should be doing'.

We went into hospital against my better judgement; my waters were artificially ruptured. Hindsight has a reputation for being a wonderful thing! As soon as you interfere with birth you're asking for problems. Birth doesn't like to be told what to do. My baby wasn't ready, and I knew it. I should have stuck to my guns, and refused consent. But I didn't. Eliza presented with shoulder dystocia. (Her shoulder got stuck coming out of the birth canal). All ten pounds and four ounces of her were put in my arms. She was blue. We ended up in NICU for a variety of reasons, which, looking back, was unnecessary; and a lot of it was to do with unacceptable mistakes made by the 'experts' at the resuscitation table.

The next few days were a steep learning curve, as we endured the world of plastic cribs, and staff that seemed hell-bent on giving every baby in sight fake milk, despite having Breastfeeding Friendly posters over all the walls.

Although many women have fed a toddler over their large belly while growing a new baby, a lot don't continue breastfeeding when finding themselves pregnant again, because, aside from books at La Leche League and other breastfeeding support groups, there's very little information available. We don't tend to see breastfeeding in pregnancy, for the simple reason that most women who are still breastfeeding after infancy, usually stop breastfeeding in public.

What does the toddler gain from breastfeeding in pregnancy? This seems to be top of the question list. As soon as most people see a kid walking, or wearing shoes, or worse, talking, they can't reconcile that with breastfeeding. A toddler has every bit as much to gain from breastfeeding as an infant.

Physically, they receive an immunological boost from <u>every</u> breastfeed. They continue to develop their jaw and facial muscles in a way that doesn't happen with bottle-feeding. Weaning before the age of two *increases the risk of illness*[12]. Breastfeeding helps a toddler adjust to life with a new sibling, by them being included in the breastfeeding process.

There is no scientific evidence that breastfeeding in pregnancy causes harm to mother or foetus.

Some people are concerned that the nipple stimulation of breastfeeding in pregnancy might lead to contractions. There is absolutely no evidence, scientific or anecdotal, to suggest labour being brought on early by this. So long as you're eating nutritious foods and resting well, there's absolutely no reason why you can't breastfeed, grow a baby and nurture your own body. If you're concerned about anaemia, please avoid resorting to a doctor's prescription for iron tablets. Apart from not being natural, they'll make you constipated, which is the last thing you need. Try dried apricots, or have a spoon of organic, unsulphured blackstrap molasses each day. Either have it off the spoon or blended with rice milk and a banana.

Natural sources of iron
Split peas
Cooked lentils
Hommous (chick pea dip)
Kidney, Adzuki, Pinto, White and Black-eye beans
Tahini
Almond butter
Uncooked quinoa
Tomatoes
Kale
Potatoes (keep the skin on!)
Broccoli
Peas
Nori seaweed
Hijiki seaweed
Prunes and dried apricots
Blackstrap molasses
Firm and regular tofu

NOTE: bread and (non herbal) tea inhibit the absorption of iron.

The Drinks Are On Me

How commonly we accept toddlers being pacified by blankies, dummies and plastic bottles, yet the situation where a child has these needs met naturally through full-term breastfeeding leads to cultural disgust.

The most obvious and natural place to gain nutrition and nurturing is at our mother's breast. Children don't forfeit their independence because they weaned naturally ~ far from it. Knowing their relationship with mother is secure, gives them a firm footing in the world. It's often quoted that breastfed children have a higher IQ than their artificially-fed peers. There's a good reason for this, which I've elaborated on in the chapter called *Who's the Dummy?*

Emotional intelligence is more important, in many ways, than intellectual strength. Our children receive many gifts from being breastfed; and certainly with more long term breastfeeding, we see that children have a higher self-esteem, and a sense of being accepted and valued. In our arms they learn intimacy, the most valuable gift for relationships. We provide them with warmth and comfort.

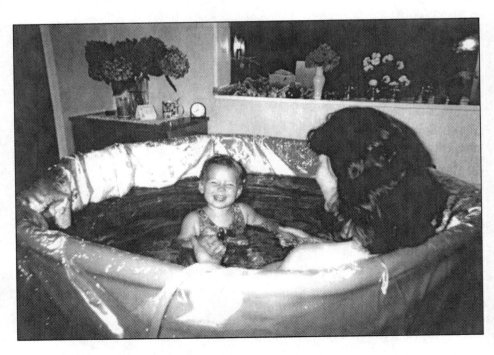

Bethany continued breastfeeding throughout my labour with Eliza, and enjoyed sharing the birthing pool.

Make mine a double!

Tandem nursing is the art of breastfeeding two children of different ages during the same time period. This doesn't always mean that you're physically nursing both children at the same time, although some women do. When a mother decides to tandem-nurse, it is because she understands that natural child-led weaning for an older child is equally as important as breastfeeding a newborn.

People who don't understand tandem nursing make inaccurate assumptions about a woman's mental state, suggesting that she's the one who needs the breastfeeding experience, as some sort of emotional crutch. Given that you can't force a child to breastfeed, it seems somewhat off the mark. Like many experiences in life, there are pros and cons. Tandem nursing is no different. Each family has to decide if it's a journey they wish to take. The decision to tandem nurse comes from a strong belief in natural weaning. If the child hasn't weaned before the birth of its sibling, then why not continue? A mother's experience of tandem nursing will be determined by the age gap between children, and her attitude to breastfeeding as a positive experience for mother and child.

Tandem nursing allows sibling love to develop, rather than jealousy. Long-term breastfeeding reduces breast cancer ~ the longer you breastfeed, the less likely you are to develop cancer[13]. It offers hydration and comfort during illness, when often no other food or drink will be accepted. Although my girls, for the most part, have always been healthy and hearty children, there were times, like when the three of us were in bed with flu or chicken pox, that all they had, or wanted, was breast milk. A woman's body is easily able to breastfeed up to about four children, so there's no need to fear that your baby might miss out on breast milk because of a nursing toddler.

One of the main disadvantages of tandem nursing stems from the common dislike amongst mothers, of breastfeeding both children at the same time. The key to tandem success seems to lie in feeding one child at a time, to avoid over-stimulating the nipples. The body is able to make milk appropriate to the needs of each suckling child. It is indeed a miracle of nature that it's able to produce age-appropriate milk for whoever is at the breast.

Coming home from hospital after Eliza's birth, we walked into our family room, which my mother had lit with candles. She played "Welcome To My World" as we entered, and had baked a beautiful plum cake for our homecoming. I wept. This is where we should have been all along. There's no better place for giving birth, and initiating breastfeeding naturally, than in the sanctuary of your own home: a place filled with love, memories and comforting smells. The reality of tandem nursing two children under two, on cue, hit me like a truck! It wasn't helped by the fact that my mother, who'd been with us for three weeks, had to fly out of the country the morning after I got home.

The Drinks Are On Me

The gift she had given, by allowing Eliza to suckle while in NICU, was priceless.

Bethany stopped eating foods completely. She lived for breast milk. At one point she looked really chubby. She was abundantly rewarded for her patient wait, with rich milk. Her experience is shared by many toddlers who've nursed through their mother's next pregnancy.

I was constantly amazed at my chubby and happy girls, and how vibrantly healthy they were. Could my breast milk really sustain two children like this? Yes indeed!

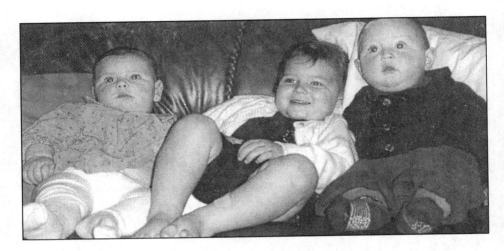

Eliza, Bethany and their friend Zachary ~ living on nothing but pure, perfect breast milk ~ audition for the Auckland sumo wrestling team!

I was never able to get them into a rhythm of sleeping in the day at the same time. They simply had different sleep needs and patterns. By evening I was exhausted. Night-time consisted of me feeding Eliza, her falling asleep, me rolling over to feed Bethany, her falling asleep, and then just about nodding off myself, only to be on duty to feed Eliza again.

I remember one night counting how often I awoke...I stopped when I got to fifty. I wanted to scream! Another night, Paul, Bethany and Eliza were all snoring. "This isn't fair! I'm the one who needs sleep."

During those early months, I was so exhausted that I wouldn't drive a car. Sometimes I think I only survived because of the love and support of an angelic man, and the local La Leche League meetings of central Auckland. And yet, despite what often seemed to be like never-ending breastfeeding sessions, I was able to nurture both of my children in a way that simply wouldn't have been possible had I prematurely forced Bethany into being weaned, or raised Eliza on bottles of fake milk.

The Drinks Are On Me

Having two children close together is exhausting for any parent if they're doing the childcare themselves, rather than passing on the job to a nanny or day care centre. Breastfeeding my girls made life easier, not harder.

I believe children wean when they're ready. Looking back, the challenges weren't because I was breastfeeding both of them, but that Paul and I lacked a sense of community around us. This nuclear set-up is wrong for families. We need aunties, sisters, grandmothers and friends around. We're not superwomen, we're not meant to do housework, cook, run errands, etc., **and** breastfeed our babies full-time. Yet we try and do it, and wonder why we find it so difficult.

With hindsight, I'd do a few things differently, to bring more peace to the parenting journey.

I'd make more time for self-nurturing, and I'd space the ages out between my children. Although it seems a nice idea to have them close in age so they can be 'friends' (never any guarantee!), I feel we short-circuit the right of a child to have all its needs met fully, by introducing another child into the situation too early.

Everyone has their own opinion on the right time to have another baby. My experience is that a toddler's needs are just as big as a baby's, and you simply can't honour both children *fully* unless there are two parents available 24/7. And how many Western families have that luxury?

I lived off an empty well, which is madness. My husband was brilliant, but he woke too with every breastfeeding ~ changing nappies in the night, then going to work before dawn to host a breakfast radio show.

He was equally exhausted, and didn't have the benefit of 'nursing hormones' to sustain him. He did have the benefit of my determination and his own sense of rightness towards what our babies needed. In many ways we both felt alienated by friends in the early days. I guess we just had unspoken expectations! We should have asked for help.

I've come to realise how different we all are. If I saw a mum who needed help or support, I'd be there despite what was going on in my own world, to help prepare meals, play with older children, clean house ~ whatever it took to make the passage of parenting easier. Let's be clear, I'm not a saint. But all of us can step out of our laziness, comfort zone ~ call it what you will, and reach out a hand to those in need.

I've learnt just how valued you feel through receiving acts of kindness. My friend Teresa stood at the end of my bed (she'd travelled an hour from her place to ours) and folded a week's worth of laundry. A little job, but so huge when your hands are already full.

A lovely lady from La Leche League, Wendy, travelled right across the city and left a lentil and tofu hotpot on our doorstep. I barely knew her, but this act of kindness filled me with tears. We can make such a difference to people's lives by small deeds. And yet, the small deeds become magnified into works of beauty because of the love behind them.

The Drinks Are On Me

Our neighbours, Jack and Jean, were pensioners with very busy lives, and yet they came and mowed our lawn and brought home-baked meals. And lovely old Hughy, God rest his soul, from across the drive... He was about 74 years old, and had an amazing, psychic ability to turn up in front of our double glass doors just when both girls had latched-on. It's impossible to be discreet with a toddler and babe both breastfeeding at the same time. "All that meat and no veg.," he'd say, shaking his head and trying his best not to smile. Cheeky beast! I never once felt his disapproval.

I'm so grateful for the support and friendship we did have. However, I recommend that good support systems are in place before birth. And again, really take time to consider the impact of the space you leave between births. Nothing can prepare you for trying to meet the different needs of two very young children.

We did continuum-style parenting on our own. It's simply not meant to be done without a community. Looking back, where we lived, in a cul-de-sac, with elderly people all around, was certainly better than it might have been. Retired people have time for young children (and mums) and are invaluable at helping to bring calm and balance to the day, even through something as simple as an afternoon chat over the garden fence.

***

At ten months, Eliza had croup. We were living on the Sunshine Coast, in Queensland, Australia, by this point. The doctor said to go straight to hospital, where Eliza would be given steroids, and be kept in overnight. We'd previously endured the torture of allowing Eliza to be given a spinal tap at six weeks, to check for meningitis, when it turned out she had nothing more than a throat infection! I wished I'd followed my intuition and just said "no". But eventually, you do learn to trust your inner voice rather than an external one, or a so-called expert. With croup, I intuitively felt that going to hospital was wrong. Instead, I went home with the girls, and to bed with Eliza. I asked Paul to keep Bethany with him while I nursed Eliza. She breastfed all night long, never letting go of the breast. In the morning there was not a trace of croup. The only medicine she'd had was non-stop (mother) love, and mother's milk.

By the time Bethany was six, she only asked to breastfeed occasionally, usually when we'd had a battle of wills or she wanted to *'be a tiny baby forever'* ~ a reaction to Eliza still breastfeeding a lot, no doubt.

Eliza, at four, breastfed most days about three to four times. It was always the first thing she asked for upon waking each day. I'm sure she dreamt about breastfeeding as well, for it to be so much in her consciousness. She'd have quite happily snuggled on my lap for hours on end if I'd had nothing else to do. She loved to know I wasn't wearing a bra. Both my children found bras to be a nuisance during breastfeeding. Some people may be challenged by this description of a child having such a tactile and pleasurable relationship with her mother's lactating breasts. My daughters' *relationship* with them was a natural and *healthy* response to being raised in an environment rich in affectional bonding.

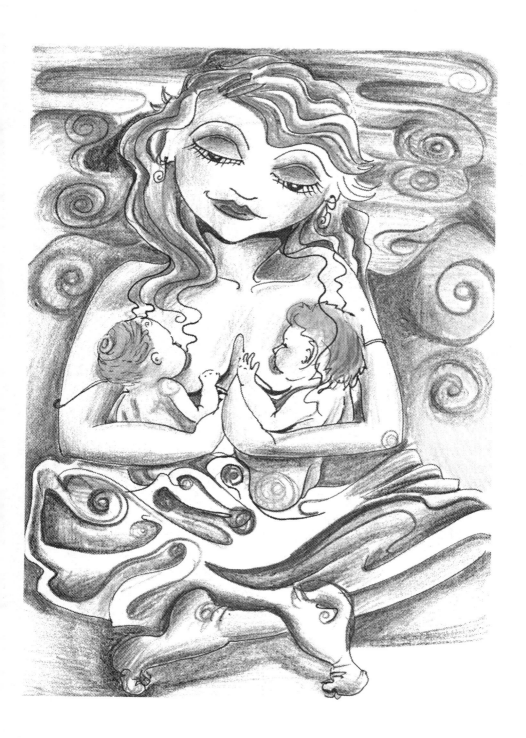

The Drinks Are On Me

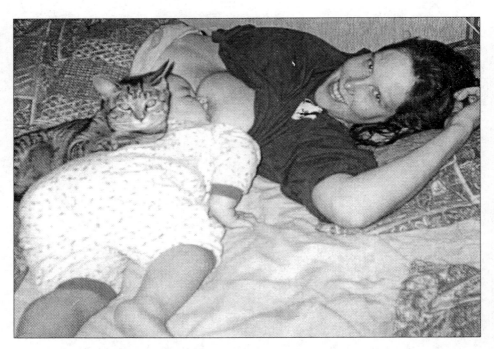

Bethany breastfeeding during my pregnancy with Eliza, accompanied by our country music feline, Catsy Pline. What is it about cats? They always find the warmest, cosiest, softest place in the home.

Why breastfeed a toddler?

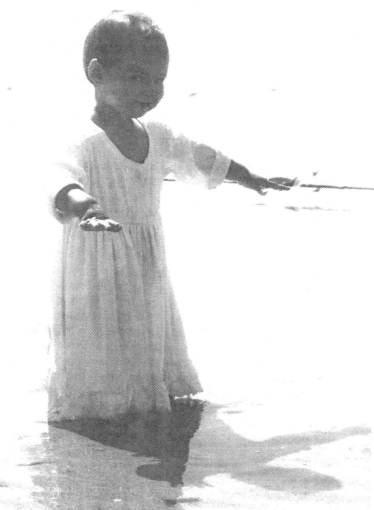

Water Princess playing on Pakiri Beach, New Zealand

The Drinks Are On Me

It's far easier raising a toddler who breastfeeds than one who relies on comfort substitutes for placation. Breastfeeding and breast milk transform toddlers when they feel overwhelmed by the environment. There simply is no need for artificial substitutes, because mother is Nature's 'security blanket'. There's no need to wash, dry-clean or sterilise a mother as we might have to with toys, blankets, dummies and so on. Breast milk is an excellent source of nutrition and energy. Feeding at the breast enhances speech, because the act of breastfeeding develops the jaw and oral muscles. During times of illness, a toddler will often refuse all food and drink. Breast milk hydrates a child when no other liquid are being taken. And for some women, the delay of menstruation because of continued nursing is often considered a bonus.

According to the World Health Organisation, breast milk provides:

100% of energy intake from 0-6 months
70% of energy intake from 6-8 months
55% of energy intake from 9-12 months
40% of energy intake from 1-2 years

Fresh foods complement the continuation of breastfeeding into toddlerhood. These percentages are based on a child having other foods. Many babies exclusively breastfeed for 12 months or more, so therefore it would still provide <u>100%</u> of their energy requirements.

Boundaries

One thing I see over and over again with mothers of breastfeeding toddlers, is the need to blame normal toddler behaviourial 'issues' on breastfeeding. Weaning doesn't take away the parent-toddler battle of will. When a toddler wants to breastfeed *all the time*, it's because he is, for the first time in his short life, engaging not only more actively in the world, but also in a new sense of who he is. He's discovering himself to be a separate entity to mother, which is all at once, fun, exciting, thrilling and downright terrifying. The child constantly needs to know mother is available for when he's reached the limit of his exploration, adventure and frustration.

All children need boundaries, and a parent's job is to provide them consistently, with compassion and love. Withdrawing breastfeeding in order to 'control' a toddler simply isn't going to work. Toddlers struggle with our modern society. We expect them to sit still, to be ignored while we take phone calls, send e-mails, have a shower, talk to a friend for hours in a coffee shop, etc.

If we were living more in accord with our biological continuum, our toddler wouldn't be relying on 'just us', or a weekly coffee group, for socialisation and as providers of opportunities to explore the world. He'd be interacting with an extended family and discovering his own boundaries in the natural world, with sticks, stones, leaves, water, etc.

Breastfeeding and breast milk transform toddlers when they feel overwhelmed by the environment.

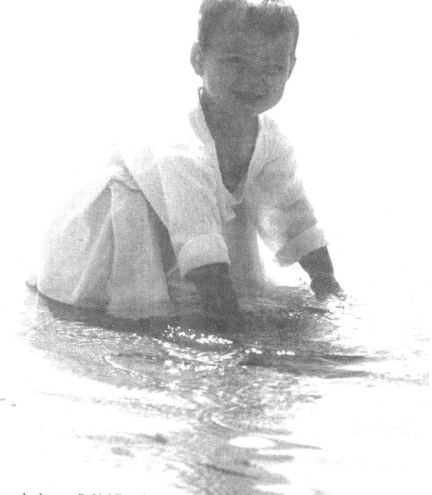

Bethany playing on Pakiri Beach, New Zealand

The Drinks Are On Me

As adults, we put ridiculously high and unrealistic expectations on toddlers, and appear to have little compassion for their needs. Many toddlers are weaned during that transformative window between the ages of two and three, oftentimes because a parent hasn't understood their child's basic needs. This abrupt weaning leaves the child confused and betrayed. A toddler needs the unconditional love of his mother more than ever.

There's a distinct difference between the breastfeeding needs of a two year old, and that of a three year old. It's almost as if a whole new person emerges in the space of twelve short months. And again, the needs change greatly between ages three and four. Without a doubt, the third year of life, between the ages of two and three, is an all-consuming period for the full-time parent of a toddler. Breastfeeding can bring huge blessings, insights and calm to what is often known as a turbulent year. A positive and healthy attitude from both parents is a vital ingredient.

Bedwetting/breastfeeding

Research into the correlation between breastfeeding and bedwetting has shown that children who were weaned from the breast before three months were *twice* as likely to wet their bed in childhood. It is considered that the neurodevelopment of the child is hindered or delayed by not breastfeeding, and this can have a profound impact on night time bedwetting[14].

Articulating the breastfeeding experience

My breasts have been called many names: bb, boobies, The Sippy Thing, booba, tit, breast, breastas, mummy juice, mama's milk, The Nips, Waking and Resting Booba, Milkior and Boobior (Two Wise Breasts at Nativity time). By the way, take it from me, tit might be easy for a toddler to say, but it's *not* a good name to have if your child is calling for it in public ~ like in a busy café. Go for something which doesn't have the same meaning, like 'money'. "Mum, money!" They'll just think your kid is gonna go far in life... which is preferable to customers spitting their cappuccino all over the table.

That my breasts have had so many names is both a reflection of the changing nature of my children and the breasts, but mostly the level of affection the children have had for them. The many children I know who've breastfed beyond infancy, have all had names of affection, and consider their mother's breasts to be their friends.

One girl, about a year after self-weaning, saw her mother getting dressed, and asked if she could 'hello' the breasts. For her, it was like witnessing the return of good friends.

Even the Buddhist Goddess Tara had her breasts named. They were Wisdom and Compassion. It beats the heck out of Resting and Waking!

No matter what time of the day or night, where we were or what we were doing, my breasts have never let me down, but they always let-down.

Breastfeeding in toddlerhood can make the terrible twos the terrific twos. Breastfeeding allows the child to have comfort during the time in their life when they're discovering they're actually a separate being to mother. They come and go, from us, the matrix, back and forward, back and forward. We provide them with so many things when we breastfeed. Security in a mother's unconditionally loving arms, drinking in liquid love, is something which lives within every cell of a child's being, and journeys with them through the rest of their life.

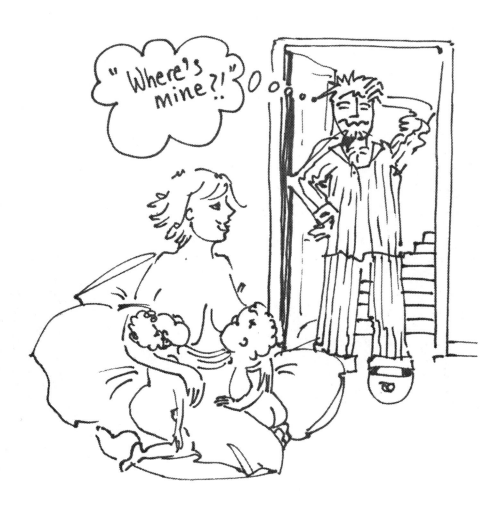

The Drinks Are On Me

*Fathers can be invaluable in supporting and nurturing
the breastfeeding relationship
between mother and child.*

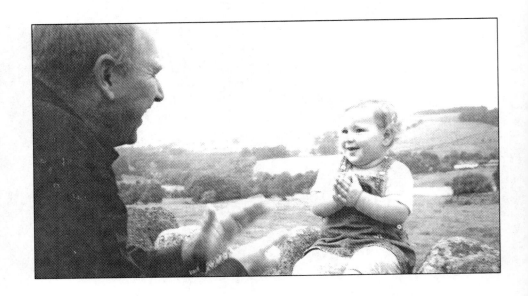

Bovine babies

In the UK, the government spends 14 pence per baby promoting breast milk. Compare this to the £20 per baby spent promoting formula milk by its manufacturers[15].

Humans have relied on breast milk throughout history. Indeed, as a species, we couldn't have come this far without breast milk. The replacement of mother's milk by formula milk in the last 60 years is but the blink of an eye in our history, yet already we see the huge consequences of our *bovine* babies. The health issues are mind boggling, and we ignore them at our peril.

During the 1950s, the breastfeeding rates in the USA dropped to a mere twenty percent (according to published figures). However, some experts in the field believe that the breastfeeding rates might have been even lower, based on anecdotal and unpublished research. So many babies who've never tasted their own mother's milk!

Thanks to the wonderful work of La Leche League and other breastfeeding organisations, the breastfeeding rate has increased. However, many mothers are still tempted to bypass breastfeeding completely. Why is that? For some mums, it's because they don't want to be 'tied down'. Tied down? It's all about perception, this mothering thing. What if we changed our attitude, and thought of our children as constant companions who've chosen us for their journey through life?

Many people often think the only difference between breast milk and fake milk is in the 'branding', a bit like the difference between Coke or Pepsi. There's a world of difference and when we truly understand why breast milk is so vital, we also recognise that it is equally as vital to be 'attached' to our children.

Cows' milk and goats' milk are designed to help calves and kids (*goat* kids) grow very quickly in a short amount of time. There's nothing in the milk's composition that suggests it was designed to grow a human baby. And yet, rather than be tied down, or work through breastfeeding challenges, or defy cultural norms, we consistently give fake milk derived from other animals. Who are we trying to kid? How long can we get away with this before there's no turning back?

Humanity is constantly evolving. It's our nature. Whether you believe in The Creation or the Big Bang theory, there's no arguing that humans are evolving. At least that's what is *meant* to be happening. The whole point of evolution is to 'get better'. To become *more* of who we are. Can we do that if we raise a new generation on something other than human milk?

Now if we take a baby, and instead of giving it the 'codes' hidden miraculously in its mother's breast milk, we give it *bovine* codes, what do you think might happen? What messages does a calf receive at a cellular level? These are the messages that children raised on calf milk are receiving!

Cow's milk makes babies grow quickly, but it can't make them grow in the way a calf grows. Something 'wants' to grow, but it can't grow any more than it has, so the potential to grow tumours occurs instead[16].

Humans are amazingly resilient. Ok, so you can raise a child on fake milk. But you can't raise it well on fake milk. No child thrives on artificial milk. If we were to take rats into a laboratory and deny them rat milk, how many generations do you think it would take before we were able to see with our own eyes, the deleterious effects of non-species milk being ingested day after day?

Humans are currently in the laboratory, but because of our long life-spans, and the relatively short time in our evolutionary history that we've not been using mother's milk, most people aren't seeing *the signs*. We've got too many other things we can blame for our lack of well-being, emotional intelligence and brain formation.

And when a few generations of fake milk-fed humans start mating with other fake milk-fed humans, we'll see the dire and probably irreversible consequences. Bet your mother never told you that...

The Formula Milk Evolution?

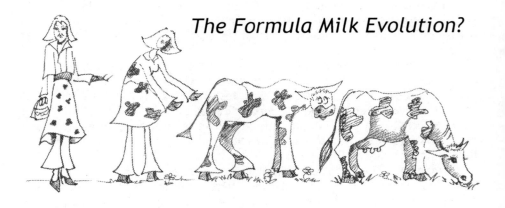

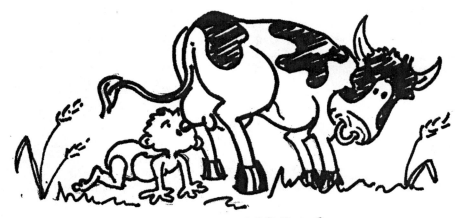

PULL THE UDDER ONE

Another consideration for infants raised on artificial milk is the risk of the water, which is added to the powder, being contaminated. Then there is the risk of contaminants within the formula. This isn't just a problem in developing countries. Water can be contaminated by many things, such as bacteria, parasites, solvents, lead, arsenic, insecticides, fertiliser nitrates, chlorine. An immature immune system simply can't cope with so much toxicity.

Unlike breast milk, which is sterile at source, it is near impossible to provide sterile formula milk, especially if you don't have safe running water, or a clean home, refrigeration, a source of heating or cleaning equipment.

It's tempting for mothers on low incomes to over-dilute the artificial milk, to make it go further. This will clearly mean the child will be short on nutrients, and eventually suffer malnutrition. It's important for mothers who choose formula milk to know that the artificial iron in it is a precursor to growing bacteria. The iron in breast milk is always appropriate to a baby's needs.

> *So many babies*
> *who've never tasted*
> *their own mother's milk!*

The Drinks Are On Me

Public Health Care

In all the literature available on breastfeeding, very little attention is given to the long-term, **life-long** benefits of breastfeeding and consequences of not breastfeeding. Babies who received very short-term breastfeeding, or none at all, have a much higher incidence in adulthood of[17]:

Depression
Poor memory
Adrenal issues
Allergies
Eczema
Obesity
Heart disease
Stroke
Osteoporosis
Multiple sclerosis
Ulcerative colitis
Crohn's disease
Poor dental structure
Breast cancer
Leukaemia
Lymphoma

Five million adults in the UK alone are affected by cardio-vascular disease. Breastfeeding in infancy drastically reduces the incidence of this in adulthood[18]. The simple, natural act of breastfeeding our children could save billions of pounds in health care both in childhood, and in adulthood.

The benefits of breastfeeding in childhood are seen for at least thirty years afterwards. These figures are based on premature weaning, so just imagine how healthy our society would be if every child had the benefit of full-term breastfeeding.

Weather girl

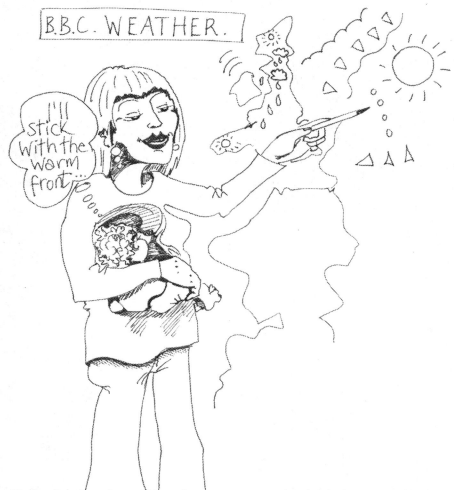

My husband reckons I'd make a great weather girl, because I have a warm front! Did you know that the temperature of breast milk is constant regardless of the weather? And that the consistency and flavour is always changing?

I have breastfed in 38 degrees Celsius on a hot Australian beach, and in below freezing snow in Northern England. I have breastfed in the humidity of Brunei and Dubai. I've breastfed during an Italian winter, and in a New Zealand kauri forest. No matter where I've breastfed, the temperature of my breast milk remained constant, and required no heating.

The Drinks Are On Me

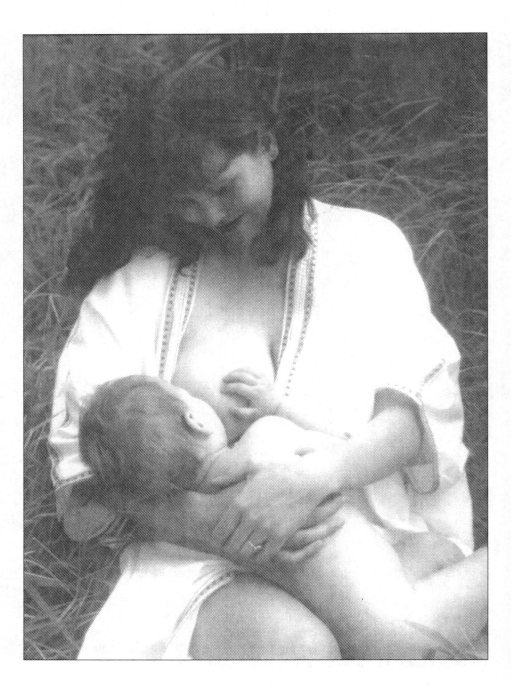

The Drinks Are On Me

"Breastfeed me NOW!"

What's the difference between feeding on demand and on cue?

Just who's in charge here? Breastfeeding on demand is considered a good thing, and it is, compared to a rigid, parent-led timetable or routine. But the language is not clear. To follow our baby's *cue*, rather than demand, shows that we're working with the baby, and that we recognise thirst or hunger, or the need for comfort, before the needs overwhelm the baby. Put simply, a baby shouldn't have to cry or scream in order for you, as a mother, to notice that she's hungry. Our cultural images show that mothers attend 'crying' babies, but this is not *nature's* way of ensuring our baby is fed well. Crying upsets the baby on many levels, and is not the best emotional or physical space in which to feed a baby, for mother or child.

How can you tell your baby is hungry? It's very simple, so simple in fact, that many parents overlook it. When your baby smacks her lips (an attuned mother can hear this even in her sleep, and will wake up), or roots out her thumb, you can be certain that hunger is demanding the baby's attention ~ and calling for yours.

Breastfeeding on demand means we're several steps *behind* a baby's cues. Breastfeeding on cue, means we're walking in step and quietly attuned. Peaceful parenting is more easily achieved when we listen to our baby's every message. Listening to her cues is easier when we co-sleep and wear her in a sling against our body. Let's put it simply: babies aren't nasty creatures ~ they always ask to breastfeed nicely first. When you don't listen, then they'll start demanding that you take notice. And rightly so!

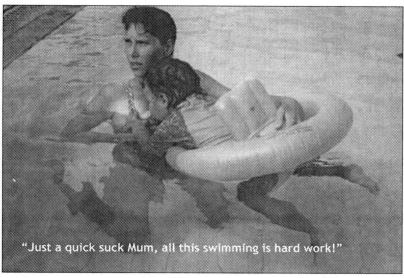

"Just a quick suck Mum, all this swimming is hard work!"

The Drinks Are On Me

A sign of a civilised society?

One third of all new mothers in the UK don't even attempt breastfeeding. This is equivalent to 200,000 babies born each year who are bottle-fed fake milk from birth. By two weeks of age, only half of all babies are breastfed. Formula-fed babies are at risk from sickness and disease, both in childhood and adulthood. They are *severely* compromised. Babies who aren't breastfed are also more likely to be abandoned by their mother[19].

There are so many excuses not to breastfeed, probably as many as there are women. And I've heard at least a hundred reasons. Some are based on ignorance and lack of breastfeeding knowledge, some on confused priorities, e.g. "I don't have time", and others are based on selfishness. The World Health Organisation and UNICEF state that over one million babies lives could be saved each year by breastfeeding[20].

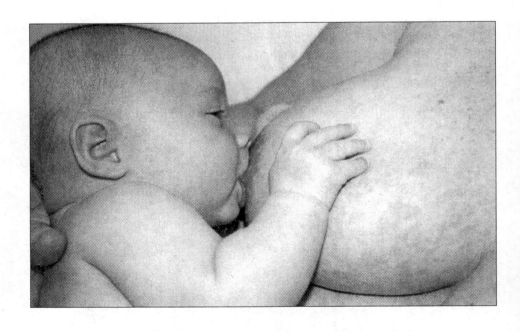

Andorra's perfect latch. Note how the lips are flanged and taking in most of the areola. This is what a baby's mouth should look like when breastfeeding.

Safety in numbers

Receiving support from other breastfeeding women isn't just about when you're having problems. Support groups exist to provide a community, to give a place to be heard, and, most importantly, to help honour a woman for being a mother ~ something considered insignificant and replaceable, in our culture.

I was recently asked if I thought there was enough support for breast-feeding women. The greatest support we can give is culturally, by eliminating our fear of seeing a child at the breast. The more normal we make breastfeeding, the less we'll hear of 'insufficient milk syndrome'.

I've had the joy of attending breastfeeding support groups in New Zealand, Australia and the UK. They were all different, but I learnt so much and always felt supported. It was humbling to get to a place some years later where I was able to provide support to other mums (even if my kids used those meetings to breastfeed the whole time).

My first experience of La Leche League was of the group in Central Auckland, New Zealand. It was during one of their coffee mornings for mums to get together and socialise, that I saw a girl of four or five breastfeeding! Can you imagine such a thing? She was spread right across her mum's lap, legs dangling right over the edge. I'd never seen anything like it. The truth is though, I wasn't disgusted, just shocked. My mind was completely stretched that day. I've always been an avid reader, but suddenly I wanted to know more about this thing I was doing day in, day out, night in, night out. I learnt so much about breast milk and breastfeeding. It's often said that we know more about how our cars work, than our bodies. Well, most humans don't know the first thing about the very food nature designed us to live on for our early years.

I attended meetings of the then Nursing Mothers' Association, in Queensland (now Association of Breastfeeding Mothers), when we moved from New Zealand to Australia.

Every breastfeeding group is different, by nature of the fact that it's made up of people with different values and beliefs. One group I went to consisted of women who wanted to know how to heat breast milk in a microwave, so they could provide expressed milk when they returned to work. I felt like a fish out of water.

When we landed in a remote part of the north of England, I went to the Lakeland LLL, and it was here, under the guidance and remarkable support of group leader Paula, that I began training to become a LLL leader and breastfeeding counsellor. At last, I truly felt like I was going to be able to help other mothers. One of the most astonishing things I learnt in my avid reading of scientific breastfeeding literature, was that the human body biologically expects to breastfeed for up to about seven years of age. Why isn't this information given out to every new mother?

The Drinks Are On Me

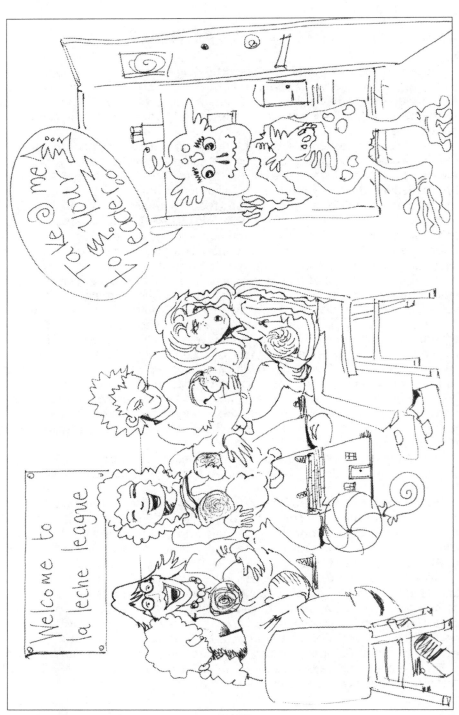

La Leche League (LLL) is an international breastfeeding support group, with local meetings held in many countries. Usually each group meets every three weeks, and discusses a breastfeeding topic. The group has a leader ~ an experienced breastfeeding mother who has undertaken LLL's breastfeeding counselling course.

Most groups have an extensive library of books and magazines to augment a mother's breastfeeding knowledge. As well as LLL, there are other breastfeeding organisations with local groups.

I can't recommend highly enough how invaluable the support is for mothers, new or experienced. If at all possible, attend during pregnancy, to increase your breastfeeding confidence and knowledge, and to become familiar with what successful breastfeeding looks like.

Breastfeeding groups are invaluable for meeting like-minded women, and are not just for mothers with breastfeeding challenges.

Such crucial information should be mandatory for a new mother. *(Indeed, what if parents had to sign an 'informed decision' document if they chose not to breastfeed, acknowledging that they fully understood the price they were paying to their own and child's health, in the short and long term; and that of future generations in their family line?)*

The research and studies backed up what I was increasingly feeling at a deep intuitive level ~ that I didn't have to impose an early curfew on my daughters' favourite activity. I did, however, feel a deep sense of sadness for every baby born who never gets to experience such bliss as being at mother's breast, or who gets a taster session, only to have it replaced with fake milk.

There are many reasons why women believe they can't breastfeed. Sometimes it's biological and other times it's a support issue. In many ways, the reasons for breastfeeding difficulties aren't much different to why some women don't appear to be able to birth without medical help. We're mammals. We're designed to breastfeed. We're designed to give birth to our babies vaginally.

When a woman finds her milk supply low or non-existent, she can be sure it isn't a 'design fault', but a symptom of the environment in which she finds herself, *and* her unconscious attitude to breastfeeding and female sexuality. This may include lack of human support, and more often than not it reflects a stressful situation around her, whether that is from others demanding her time and energy, or because of her recovery from a medicalised birth. Women should never underestimate the impact of an 'interfered with' birth. It changes our ability to parent naturally. It doesn't make it impossible by any means, but it can make it harder. Lack of information and support can inhibit the breastfeeding relationship.

Breastfeeding is very much a mind/body synergy. For our breasts to produce milk for our babies, we need to be mentally present and emotionally willing. Support for breastfeeding is available to all women, however it doesn't sit on most people's doorsteps. We have to actively seek it out. Ideally, we'd do so before birth. Like birth, when we initiate breastfeeding, it should ideally be in a quiet, calm and homely atmosphere, without an audience.

We have to ask ourselves the obvious question, "do I want to breastfeed?" We have to truly *want* to breastfeed, rather than take a lackadaisical approach. It's a choice with no half-way mark. We prepare ourselves for breastfeeding by seeking out support, information and like-minded people ~ ideally breastfeeding mums, as they are the *experts* on their breastfed children, and can help us to hear our own expert selves. Our human nature determines that we will breastfeed. To choose otherwise, consciously or subconsciously, is not an easy decision, and has consequences for years to come, for mother, father, child, grandchildren, great grandchildren and so on, through the generations. It can be hard to breastfeed through challenges if we've not received accurate information. It doesn't make it impossible though.

The Drinks Are On Me   ~ 110 ~

It's too easy for people in the natural birthing/breastfeeding world to succumb to judgement, and turn their backs on people who choose, consciously or otherwise, to have unnecessary c-sections, or use formula milk. Our job is to step into the arena and bring our knowledge and experience for others to share; but we must always come from a place of compassion and sisterly love. It never hurts to remind ourselves, that in different circumstances, with different people in our lives, our path may have been completely different. Likewise, it's just as important not to hide the truth about breastfeeding because we fear offending someone.

When we are surrounded by people who share our outlook, we feel reassured, and our confidence in life choices increases.

It's not uncommon for women who begin breastfeeding, to start feeling uncomfortable when everyone around them is bottle-feeding. We choose whether to live socially isolated lives so that we don't feel uncomfortable, or make positive choices to search out like-minded mums.

Reasons given for stopping breastfeeding
The main reasons women give for stopping breastfeeding are:
Nipple pain from baby not being latched-on properly *(avoidable and remediable)*.
Pressure by health-care worker *(always listen to your own voice)*.
Pressure by their partner *(usually based on jealousy, insecurity and lack of breastfeeding knowledge because they weren't breastfed. Explain that a successful breastfeeding relationship does not exclude him)*.
A misguided belief in low milk supply, and lack of information on how the demand and supply system of breastfeeding works *(educate yourself)*.
Mother going back to work and not understanding that she can still breastfeed *(learn how to express milk, and remember you can breastfeed mornings, nights and weekends)*.

> *Snow flakes*
> *are one of nature's*
> *most fragile things*
> *but just look what they can do*
> *when they stick together.*
>
> **Verna Kelly**

The Drinks Are On Me

You may feel in a minority group, but what a *powerful* minority you're in if you choose breastfeeding. You'll become stronger, more powerful and make continued appropriate choices for your child in your parenting. It's inevitable that by standing strong and true to one's self that we draw others into our circle.

It's important we don't ever apologise for choosing to breastfeed. Don't undermine yourself. You're a living picture to your children. If you feel unworthy, your kids will copy that. Our self-esteem has a habit of following us throughout our lifetime. Bring yourself to mothering in a spacious, wholesome and respectful way.

It's not uncommon to hear a non-breastfeeding mother say that women who breastfeed make bottle-feeders feel guilty. Guilt is a 'thought', *not* a feeling, and the thought is a *choice*. Guilt is invaluable at guiding us through life and letting us know when we're *compromising*. I don't think it is something we should ever fear. It lets us know when we're off the path. What is important is how we choose to experience and acknowledge the guilt.

The truth is, though, that the anti-breastfeeding community is so large and strong within our culture that those who follow Mother Nature sound like roaring lions for praising the qualities of the breastfeeding way. Because we believe so strongly in the rightness and common sense of breast milk, it's almost inevitable that we come across as zealots. But, who better to advocate breastfeeding than a breastfeeding mother?

Bottle-feeding, although the most common choice, isn't based on common *sense*; it's completely based on fear and lack of knowledge. That fear can come from many factors, such as feeling tied down, modest about your body, fear that a partner won't find you sexy, peer pressure and ignorance of breastfeeding and its myriad benefits.

Bottle-feeding our children artificial milk lets everyone down in numerous ways. Firstly, it's difficult for the baby to digest. Parents wrongly assume it's good for the child because they "sleep so well" after a feed. They are, in fact, suffering digestive *exhaustion,* as their little body tries to break down curds of milk designed for a rapidly growing calf. It compromises our children's health and brain potential. Bottle-fed babies are at an increased risk of long-term and acute or chronic respiratory illnesses, such as pneumonia or asthma.

It takes a huge toll on the environment (production, transport, land for grazing cattle), and involves huge amounts of money on advertising and promotion.

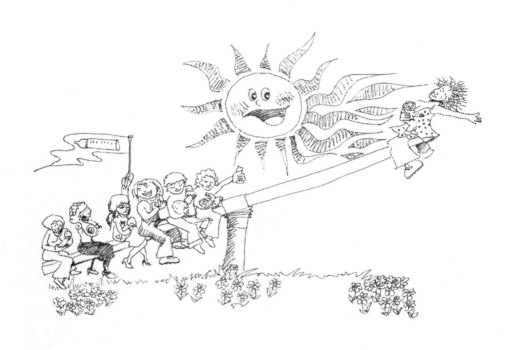

Other risks:
Contamination of artificial milk (either while being made in the home, or initially, in the factory)
Ear infections which often lead to prescriptions for antibiotics
Tooth decay from artificial sugars
SIDS
Dietary allergies
Skin allergies
Respiratory allergies
Illness when the water to formula ratio is incorrect

Babies fed on artificial milk are **ten** times more likely to end up in hospital by the age of 12 months, compared to their breastfed peers[21]. It's not a random coincidence, it's a massive warning sign that our culture ignores at its peril.

The Drinks Are On Me

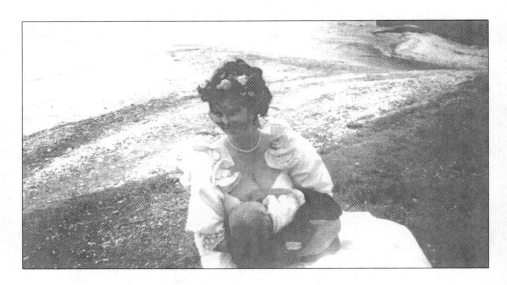

Breastfeeding Bethany on my wedding day.
Green Bay, Auckland, New Zealand.

Breastfeeding underground

Why are we scared to breastfeed in public?

A few hundred years ago it was the cultural norm in the UK to breast-feed for several years. Queen Victoria passed a law to make sure that bar-ing breasts was not done in public! This led to breastfeeding becoming very much an out of sight activity.

By the 1950s, eight out of every ten babies in the USA were artificially fed from birth. Artificial milks became a sign of wealth, and usurped Mother Nature's perfect milk as a symbol of status. This has become the norm in Third World countries too. If you're concerned about breastfeeding politics, look no further than the book *Breastfeeding Matters* by Maureen Minchin. Clearly, if you read this book before choosing bottle-feeding, then you can *honestly* say you made an informed choice.

It's no coincidence that the move away from natural infant feeding has coincided with the increase in medically managed births. More and more women are giving their innate power to birth and breastfeed over to others.

When we have no option but to breastfeed, we, as mothers, manage to find ways through problems and challenges, just as we would with child-birth. If you had no option but to breastfeed your baby because otherwise it would die, what would your choice be? Silly question? Perhaps we encour-age slow death by not breastfeeding? Perhaps the baby's body is screaming out for us to listen, by developing eczema, asthma, allergies, constant ear infections, thumb sucking, etc.

Countries which maintain strict guidelines around the promotion of for-mula milk have much higher breastfeeding rates. Commercial power eats at our inner knowing.

We can't, however, sit back and blame the multi-nationals because they offer us artificial milk. Like every other aspect of our lives, we have to take full responsibility for our choices and consequent actions. Life, with its busyness, tempts us with the ways and means of short-circuiting 'time'. We use any number of excuses to put our baby onto artificial milk.

I've breastfed in places of worship, in supermarket queues, on the beach, in forests, a bank manager's office (tandem nursing! It was the only way I could get a conversation without the girls hijacking it), buses, trains, cars, planes, driving to my wedding, at my wedding, in the swimming pool, library. We don't need anyone's permission to breastfeed our babies in pub-lic, ever. It's the ultimate in human rights abuse to deny a baby the right to feed from its mother at any time it needs to. That we allow ourselves to be bullied into breastfeeding in toilets, of all places, is tragic.

The Drinks Are On Me

I don't know about you,
But I'd never eat in a public loo,
where people come to poo!

~ W. Shakespeare

Well, maybe not Will's wise words, but how many women 'allow' themselves to be bullied into breastfeeding their baby in what is no less than a sewage pit?

We can provide great support every time we see a breastfeeding woman, by making eye contact and smiling. Invite breastfeeding women into the public arena and out of public toilets by acknowledging that they're doing a great job!

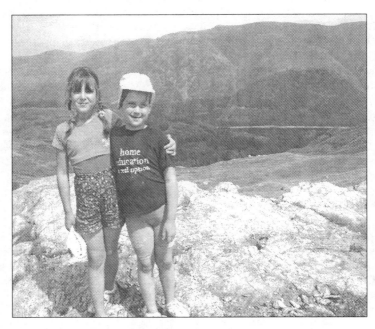

Bethany and Eliza, growing out of breastfeeding and climbing mountains in England's Lake District.

Coming out of the closet

I had an e-mail from a researcher at an independent tv production company in London, which was interested in doing a documentary on extended breastfeeding. A cameraman came with her to Cumbria, and did some taster filming with myself and a few other mums, who were breastfeeding toddlers.

Apparently, I was so normal looking, whatever that means, on the taster filming, that the production company got the commission because someone in charge couldn't believe anyone not wearing muslin clothing, hair in braids, and socks in sandals would choose this path. How wrong they were. It's clear that women from *all* walks of life choose to breastfeed their children until they've had their fill.

By the time the commission came, however, I decided that actually I didn't want to put myself in the public eye and risk the inevitable consequences of being misrepresented. But I hadn't counted on hearing from Katie Buchanan. How dare she be so lovely?

Katie was the producer, and was so kind, genuine and open minded ~ not to mention supportive, that I found myself reconsidering; and before long, we had cameras and an all-woman team documenting our unusual, by western standards, breastfeeding story. Eliza seemed to reconnect with breastfeeding in ways I'd never even thought of, and her final feed was delayed by about 8 months! The whole experience of being talked about in the national media magnified for her the fact that something precious was finishing in her life.

She soon lost the sucking reflex, due to infrequent feeding. Eliza started to feel cheated. It's unfortunate really, because had we not been involved in the filming, she'd have weaned without giving it any conscious thought. (This is not to be confused with a nursing strike, or breast refusal, which is something a mother <u>can</u> help her child with, given it usually happens a lot earlier than with natural weaning, and often happens after the mother has gastric trouble, and the breast milk changes drastically to release the toxins.)

One thing I hadn't realised, was how few women actually know about the sucking reflex and that all children will self-wean at some point. In the documentary, I used the end of a pear and my grasping fingers, to illustrate how the sucking reflex works, and how it stops working. This seems to me a vital piece of information, which should be standard in any support on breastfeeding; and yet, all the weaning literature revolves around foods to give our children in lieu of breast milk.

By taking part in Extraordinary Breastfeeding, I had only ever hoped to make a difference. It was gob-smacking to see it covered so dramatically in all forms of media; and it really rattled the country that children who could talk, wear shoes and actually articulate their breastfeeding experience, could be so eloquent in their joy of it.

The Drinks Are On Me

It's fair to say many, many people were utterly repulsed, and it isn't just because we don't have a cultural framework, a visual image of full-term breastfeeding; it's because these people were denied the experience, and have no *cellular concept* of such intimate, non-sexual giving and receiving.

It challenges their whole way of life, and because the mother-child bond and feeding are so fundamental to humanity's survival, it's far easier to dismiss them outright, rather than give them any conscious thought or objective consideration.

After the documentary was aired on Channel Four in February 2006, thousands of families finally felt they could speak out about their experiences. I was inundated with letters, e-mails and phone calls from parents of children around the four year old mark, who were wondering how they'd wean their child. They didn't know about the sucking reflex either, and felt so grateful to learn about natural weaning.

Bootleg copies of the documentary found their way around the world. It really was funny to receive e-mails from people from the furthest corners of the globe, even in non-English speaking countries, all united in the understanding that although full-term breastfeeding isn't common in our culture, it's natural. More than a year later, I still receive e-mails from mums, dads and breastfeeding professionals, who've been touched by the fact I was willing to speak up about this important aspect of breastfeeding. I've been amazed at how many full-term breastfeeding mums are in existence, all hiding in the closet, in our western culture.

The phone never stopped ringing. Tv, radio and newspapers in the US, Germany and Korea all wanted a 'bit' of me. There comes a point, though, where you have to say "no", regardless of how much you want to educate and support other mums. I was badly misrepresented by many publications, whose articles were then syndicated around the world. When the deep desire to educate families ends up being *sensationalist fodder*, you do lose heart and feel there must be other, better, ways to spread the vital truth about breastfeeding.

A chord was touched with the public. What was it that caught people's fascination? I hadn't eaten someone. I wasn't a cannibal, and neither was my child. I was feeding her the food created specifically for her body for the amount of time her brain needed breast milk to develop optimally. Was my way of parenting an absolute threat to modern life? Was it so primal that it unhinged people?

I was struck by the number of questions people had about full-term breastfeeding. It seemed they just didn't know where else to go for information. One day, might we look back upon enforced weaning as something barbaric?

Some snippets from the Extraordinary Breastfeeding documentary are now being seen on the internet via YouTube. There's no stopping freedom of information! www.youtube.com Enter 'extraordinary breastfeeding' in the search bar.

The Drinks Are On Me

It's at mother's breasts that we prepare for intimate relationships in our adult lives. If we, as adults, have never had this sort of relationship it will seem like a foreign language, and we'll not be able to recognise it, so we'll dismiss it outright. We'll find all sorts of reasons to tear down *any* model of unconditional love that we see.

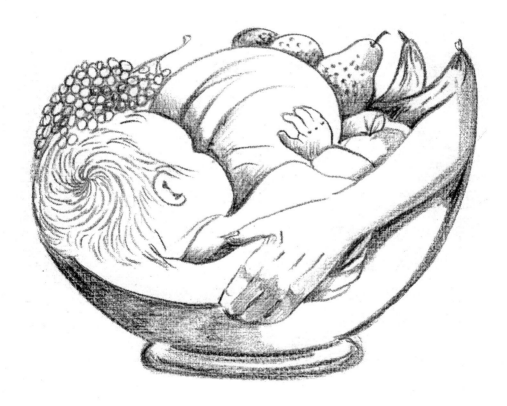

A breast a day
keeps the doctor away

The Drinks Are On Me

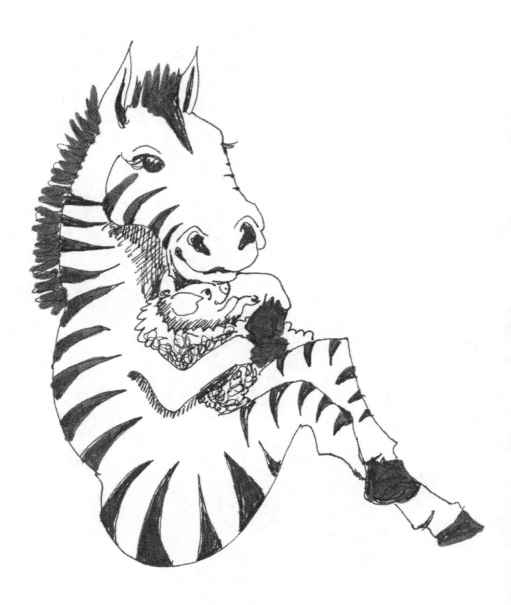

Zebras breastfeeding piglets, pigs nursing hedgehogs, cows breastfeeding humans...whatever next?

The milk bar

In my party girl days, when I used to drink milkshakes made from cow's milk, rather than rice or soya milk, my flat mate and I would head to the local milk bar and try to dull the thump in our heads ~ a nasty consequence of too much fun the night before. There were loads of flavours to choose from, my favourite being banana or mint.

I don't know why, but we never thought to ask if it was cow's milk. I mean, it could have been rat milk, camel milk, pig milk, bat milk, dolphin milk, mouse milk, cat milk.

Why is it universally 'ok' to have cow, goat or sheep milk to drink, or buffalo milk to make mozzarella, but gut-turning to think I might pour some pig milk into a glass for your morning tea? The odds are, though, given a choice, most people would take milk from another mammal before they'd *dare* to drink milk from their own species!

I find the collective psychology of society's repulsion to a lactating woman absolutely fascinating. That we readily reject the milk of our own species ,but, daily, fill our fridges with milk designed to make a calf grow *very* quickly ~ and from a mum with poo sliding down her backside and onto her udder, which then has to be pasteurised to *protect* us, well it's all a bit odd really. Some of us were brainwashed with tv adverts that had a catchy theme song "milk, a natural part of life". Yep, milk is natural ~ when it's from our mum and not a cow. And yes, natural when a calf has cow's milk.

For the record, piglets *love* pig milk. Actually, they love their mummy's milk as much as human babies love human milk from their mums. Funny that. Must be something in it.

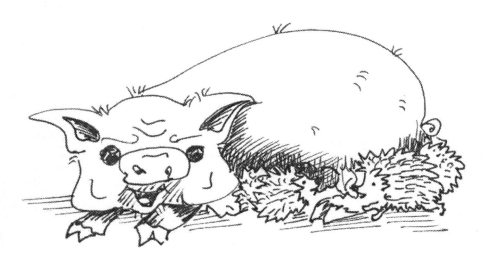

The Drinks Are On Me

I came across a woman a few years ago who was planning to set up an exhibition of women's breast milk for the public to taste samples. How amazing. I don't know if it went ahead, but exhibitions like this could be held around the world. We'd get so much more of a sense of the different compositions of breast milk: morning milk; afternoon milk; milk from a vegetarian mummy; or a mum who lives off curries; or what about colostrum? That would have to be Liquid Gold Special! And then there's Thirst Quencher (foremilk) and Tummy Filler (hindmilk). We'd learn why some women think their milk looks thin and then mistakenly give up breastfeeding, believing formula milk to be more filling.

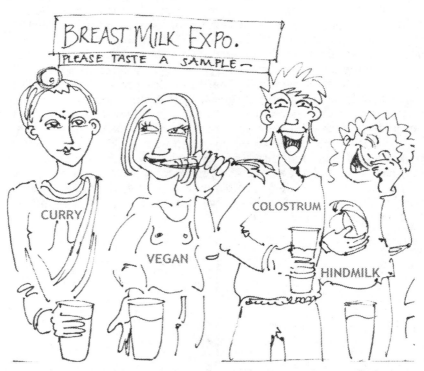

When Bethany was younger, my mum suggested I give her some bottled water, because we were going through a hot summer. Had I not already begun to study breast milk, I may well have done so. Instead, I kept letting her breastfeed whenever she wanted to, *knowing* that her thirst would always be quenched.

It's interesting how little water adults drink, and how often people reach for food thinking they're hungry, rather than thirsty. I wonder if, as children, we'd been allowed to breastfeed full-term, we might, in adulthood, recognise the difference between thirst and hunger?

The Drinks Are On Me   ~ 122 ~

Hands off my breasts!

The sexuality of breastfeeding

When I worked at the Hills Montessori School, we did a session with the children each week about body awareness, specifically to help identify any of them who had been physically or sexually abused. One of the songs we taught the children had lyrics along the lines of "My body's nobody's body but mine, You run your own body, let me run mine."

It's not unusual for women to arrive at breastfeeding and feel uncomfortable with the whole process, even when done in private. Given that statistics reveal one in four women has been sexually abused as a child, it's not surprising that we have issues around our sexuality. The little girl within never leaves us, no matter how much grey hair we grow, or how many wrinkles line our face, or stretch marks crepe our tummy. If she's been hurt, demeaned, troubled or condemned, she walks, wounded, everywhere with us through life, until such time as we consciously heal the pain and shame.

All aspects of becoming and being a mother involve our sexuality, and it's easy to confuse previous bad sexual experiences with good sexual feelings. Sometimes these are subconscious, and so we're simply not aware of what's driving us. My own experiences with men who should have known better than to touch a young girl, led me to creating a birth that would ensure I was not 'violated' again by a man (disguised as a doctor and wielding tools to interfere with me).

With Bethany, I chose to give birth in a birth pool. Doing so, in addition to having a midwife supportive of natural birthing, meant that I created a physical space around me while I underwent the most 'sexual' experience of my life. We're never more vulnerable, or as open, physically and spiritually, as we are when we give birth vaginally. Because of the way I *chose* to give birth, where I was in control of my body, and the space around me, I released a childhood of sexual abuse. Had I made different choices, it's possible I may well have ended up recreating a situation where someone else was in control of my body.

Some women need counselling to overcome issues that they might have with their nipples, or indeed other parts of their body. Others simply avoid dealing with it at all, and put their baby straight on a bottle. Sadly, the baby misses out on one of life's most beautiful and necessary gifts, and the mother misses out on an opportunity to heal, as well as discovering the absolute joy and pleasure which come from breastfeeding.

The consequences of childhood sexual abuse manifest in many areas of your reproductive life, not just an aversion to having a child suckle on your breasts. You may feel so scared to give birth that your body closes down, and you end up with a caesarean, or needing a ventouse or forceps to pull the baby out.

The Drinks Are On Me

It can contribute to increased rates of Post Natal Depression, because we've just gone through an incredible sexual experience (birth), and 1.) not been able to articulate all that emerged within our being as every cell within responded to our 'creation'; and 2.) not had the experience validated by our culture.

If we don't heal these issues before or during birth or breastfeeding, the *Great Celestial Amplifier* will just go on getting louder, and can manifest in other ways, such as heavy and painful periods, hysterectomies, menopausal symptoms. And when we finally cut away all our reproductive organs in an attempt to silence the noise our body makes, then we'll hear noises elsewhere. We can't hide from our unresolved issues. Somewhere, somehow, they'll surface.

Many breastfeeding mothers don't show an interest in sex for some time after birth. If birth has been experienced as painful or traumatic, it's logical that we'd not want to risk repeating that again in a hurry!

On the other hand, if a woman has birthed easily, which is usually a consequence of conscious conception by *both* parents, a breastfeeding mother may be more likely to match her lover's sexual desire.

Our hormones are funny things, with a language all of their own. When we learn to understand this language, then everything starts to make sense. The Greek meaning of hormone is *messenger*. And the hormones literally send messages from our brain through our body and back again.

Hormonally, the message most women receive after birthing is that they have had their 'fill'.

Women can find it emotionally painful to reject their husband's advances after childbirth. They want to join in with him sexually, to express their love; but physically (remember the hormones?), they're receiving and giving different messages.

Something relatively new in human history is the advent of the bottle-fed father. Remember back in the 1950s, we had a generation of bottle-fed babies? In the USA, only **two** out of every ten babies ever breastfed. How do we justify virtually a whole country not receiving love through mother's milk? There will come a time in our history, when we shall consider this one of the greatest crimes against humanity.

Now we have a few generations of men who've been bottle-fed. By not having had their needs met as infants, these men are stimulated, unconsciously, by seeing their wives breastfeed. How is the mother to respond? After all, we *are* sexual beings even when we lactate, but sexuality has many layers to it. A man will almost certainly be seeing the breasts as erogenous.

Those men who had their needs fully met in infancy (which these days is very rare in our culture) won't just focus on the breasts, but see the whole of their wife's body as erotic.

The birth of our children is an opportunity for men to heal their primal experiences too.

The ghost memory of their own mother can be finally given the freedom to leave, and their lover's body can be related to in a healthy, rather than obsessive, way.

One of the noticeable differences between bottle-feeding and breast-feeding is that at the breast we learn the give and take of a relationship. Our mother is a source of nourishment.

I watched a woman bottle-feeding her baby today. The baby was lying down in the pram, the mum standing with her back to him and looking away. They had no body contact whatsoever: and absolutely *no* eye contact. Where is the maternal nourishment to be found in such a scenario? Both mother and child miss out on the 'love' hormone which is produced by breastfeeding. Feeding can become a chore, rather than a pleasurable act of bonding.

We cannot relate or imprint ourselves on an inanimate object such as a bottle or dummy. They don't emote, or receive our baby's smile, or say "I love you".

Some breastfeeding women satisfy their partner by allowing him to nurse alongside their baby. When I said this on the breastfeeding documentary, there was outrage. Why, I don't know. Men the world over have been sucking on women's breasts since time began. Why is it suddenly so incomprehensible that he might also do it while his partner is lactating? If sucking on a lactating breast is taboo, then surely *any* sexual contact during lactation should be?

It's interesting to note that the men who are 'allowed' into the sacred sphere of a mother's lactating breasts realise they're not in competition for their partner's love, that they're friends with their child, and don't feel neglected or have to 'act out' in immature ways to seek attention. When a man's needs have been met like this, women tend to be comfortable in a way that they aren't when men grab at their breasts as if deeply deprived. Perhaps we'd see less incidence of adultery if men didn't feel so rejected, initially by their mother, and again by their lover. Just as we have an inner girl within, so too do men (no matter how old, grumpy, or grey haired!) have a little boy inside, more often than not crying out for attention.

The elevation of breasts in our culture as solely sexual objects, is out of proportion to other aspects of our being. It distinctly shows how out of touch with nature we've become, culturally.

Breasts have two purposes: for the nourishment/health of our children; and for erotic pleasure. As mothers, both our babies and partners are interested in them. Because they utilise the same hormones, they're not necessarily activities which can be compartmentalised. It's here that people *mistakenly* confuse the bi-functional aspects of our breasts with incest.

Breastfeeding is a sexual experience, but it isn't to be confused with sexual intercourse. Nature designed it so that breastfeeding would indeed be a pleasurable activity for mother and child.

The Drinks Are On Me

Why else would the same hormones be involved as with love-making? Because we're engaging in an *act of love* with our baby. This is nothing to be frightened of, and it doesn't mean there is anything 'wrong' with you. Those who conclude you might be perverted for enjoying breastfeeding have more to worry about than you do!

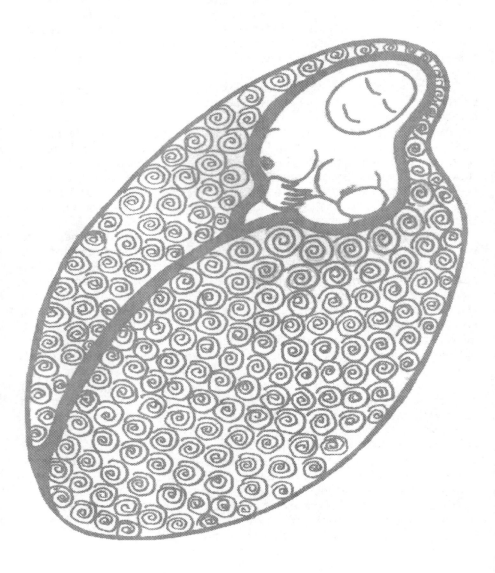

A holistic approach to sexuality

To many people the word sexuality is synonymous with sexual intercourse. This is very limiting, and makes explanation of the hormones and their impact on breastfeeding a rather challenging task! But I'll try anyway...

Sexual energy is nothing more than a *creative surge* running through our body. It *can* be channelled into sex, but is equally happy when channelled into creative pursuits like cooking a meal, tending a flower garden, painting a picture, writing a letter, singing a song and nurturing another living creature. A breastfeeding woman who has what might be described as sexual feelings, could, under the narrow-minded and misinformed dictates of our cultural thinking, feel there's something wrong with her as the hormone responses are triggered in breastfeeding. The hormones produced for love-making, and, indeed, for falling in love, are also the same ones manufactured by the body in orgasm, birth and breastfeeding. This is groovy Mother Nature at her best, showing how clever she is, so don't knock her! Multi-tasking isn't just a human skill.

Our reproductive energies are powerfully creative. To make a baby is a work of art like no other. The hormones of love and sexuality which weave their way tightly through all aspects of our lives, are designed to nurture and nourish us from cradle to grave. So why on Earth would we want to hide or denigrate such a powerful force for good? Holistic sexuality also involves recognising that the most intimate relationship we can ever have is with *ourselves*. An ideal partner is a joy, but not a necessity. By understanding, loving, caring, and most importantly, honouring our vast and multi-faceted sexual nature, we have a healthy relationship with self, that brings healing to many people.

Sex itself becomes harmful and dangerous when limited to domination, guilt, unmet needs in childhood, and shame. One of the most powerful aspects of healthy sex is when orgasm becomes an experience throughout the whole body, rather than just in the genitals. It's felt by both partners, and it involves more than just the physical being. There is no sense of separation. In many ways, the energy of a healthy and mature sexual relationship can be likened to a successful breastfeeding relationship. It's about giving and receiving, yin and yang, ebb and flow.

The Drinks Are On Me

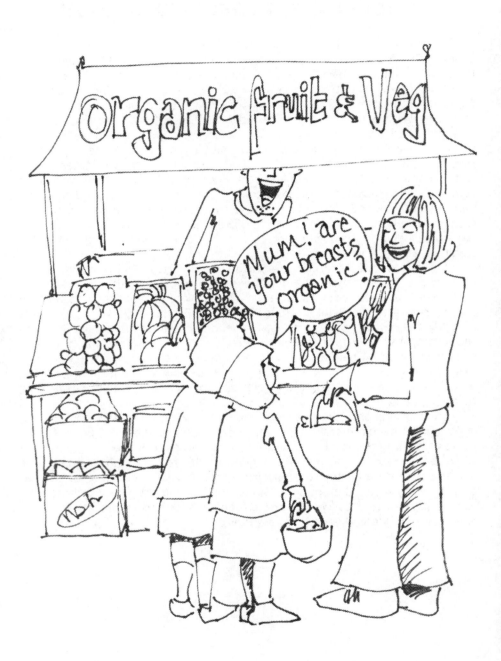

Are your breasts organic?

When Bethany was five years of age, she asked me if my breasts were organic. The latest propaganda against breastfeeding, probably put forward by no less than the infant formula companies themselves, is that there are toxins in breast milk! Not sure where they're keeping the cows and goats these days to keep them toxin free, but this argument should <u>never</u> be used to stop a woman breastfeeding. If anything, it's a huge call for humanity to clean up its environmental act!

Here's my take on it: toxins are an inevitable consequence of 21st century living. Even the poor old polar bears, who don't know the first thing about bleach, computers and plastics, are suffering ridiculous levels of toxicity.

Breast milk from your body is designed for *your* baby, and will help him to deal with environmental toxins ~ even those within your breast milk. It's a living food with so many amazing components, that to suggest not feeding it to children because their mother's body contains toxins, is the height of ignorance. The media should be using their column inches and air time to educate *everybody* how to live in ways which will reduce toxic overloads for all of us.

If we're concerned about toxins in breast milk, then we should, equally, if not more so, be concerned about the toxins our baby receives in utero. If they're in your body, then these toxins are in the environment which is creating and growing your baby.

Due to the technology used, it's much easier for scientists to test for toxins in breast milk than it is to test in cow or goat milk. We should bear this in mind when being told that there are fewer toxins in artificial milk made from cow or goat! Artificial baby milk contains things such as beef tallow and sunflower oil, and may be contaminated with pesticides, dioxins or other toxins. Levels of salmonella, aluminium and lead have been found in some brands of formula.

Foods for lactating mums

Being a breastfeeding mum means we have to take care of ourselves in a more conscious way than we might have before having a child. Keeping our fluid levels up and maintaining our energy are the keys to feeling balanced.

As someone who eats a plant-based diet, I kept my iron up by taking Floradix (a fruit-based liquid iron supplement), dried apricots and organic blackstrap molasses, as well as an abundance of raw, leafy green vegetables. A little of these each day is more than enough. If your doctor suggests iron tablets, run a mile! Constipation is not a visitor your body ever needs... Water should be the number one thing you reach for when thirsty, followed by home-made, fresh fruit and vegetable juices, and herbal teas. Eating foods which are grown without chemicals or pesticides will reduce your intake of toxins.

The Drinks Are On Me

Huge amounts of water and fertiliser are utilised in the growing of soya. In many cultures, forests are the number one source for food, providing ample nuts, fruits, herbs, leaves, fungi and roots. And, of course, countless insects, birds and animals rely on these forests too. Do we, in western culture, have a right to feed our babies on soya or cow's milk, at the cost of taking away food sources which would feed countless other people's children[26]? Twelve and a half square metres of precious, irreplaceable Mexican rainforest are destroyed to make a mere one kilogram of infant fake milk. There are no manufacturing products needed to provide a baby with breast milk. Formula milk involves the creation of toxins in providing packaging, such as tin, plastic and paper. The figures for how much un-recycled tin gets thrown out from formula milk cans are staggering.

One way to imagine the huge volume of waste created is to consider the number of babies in the USA who feed off fake milk. In just one year, the number of tins thrown out could circle our Earth one and a half times. This, from just one country!

Water is a precious resource. Man-made toxins are dumped almost everywhere. More than half of all surface water in the USA, for example, contains pollutants used in mainstream agriculture. Combine the contaminated water from this with the water used to make up the infant formula, and your baby is not off to a very good start in terms of health. Formula is relatively expensive, and so, in poor families, it's often diluted more than the instructions suggest, so that they can make the milk 'go further'. Breathing in fresh air becomes a thing of the past when we examine how much air pollution is created from the production of fake milk. This comes in various forms, such as methane gas from cows, from the production of the electricity used in the manufacture of formula, and the disposal of everything associated with the milk's packaging and use ~ bottles, teats, plastic, tin, paper labels and advertising/promotion.

Huge factories are required to make artificial milk and the equipment needed to transport and consume it. How far has the milk in your local supermarket had to travel? Has it been transported from New Zealand to the UK, or Ireland to the US? Does it say, 'grown locally'? And do you know that the modern-day version of a mother's nipple ~ a teat or dummy ~ takes anything up to 450 years to decompose in a landfill? When people no longer have the luxury of dumping their rubbish in a landfill, because there's no space left, will they be prepared to 'store' the leftovers from parenting in their own back yard? Imagine if all this money and energy went, instead, into making the world a better a place for our children and their children? Being aware of aggressive advertising techniques by multi-nationals, and raising awareness of the formula industry, is best achieved through widespread communication of these facts.

Breastfeeding is not only free, it doesn't involve the destruction of forests, erosion of soil and pollution from transportation. Breastfeeding is not connected to climate change. The impact of breastfeeding will not be visibly seen in landfills 300 years from now, or three minutes from now. It doesn't involve the use or abuse of any animal.

Breast milk is a natural, renewable, environmentally-safe resource. Breast milk does not contaminate, and needs no production, packaging, transport, preparation or disposal.

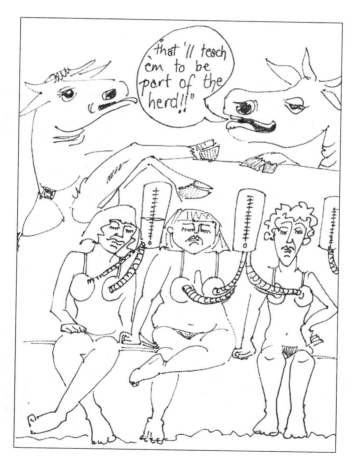

Revenge of the cows
Mummy's milk for calves

The Drinks Are On Me

Weaning

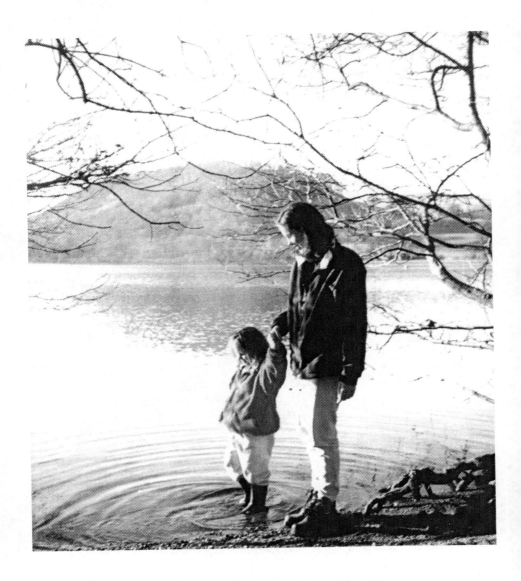

Bethany and Veronika ~ Winter in the Lake District, Cumbria UK.
Breastfeeding, too, has seasons. Child-led weaning is natural, peaceful, and, like the letting go of Autumn leaves, a season which eventually comes to pass.

When does weaning begin?

*"I've heard it called extended breastfeeding.
I just fed them long enough to really fill up their hearts,
and because (mother-led) weaning is an act of oral and emotional force."*
~ Sammy Kunina, author, Revolution Within

Weaning begins the second we introduce anything into our baby/child's mouth that isn't breast milk. More emphasis should be given to the slow, delicate and *conscious* introduction of food, rather than how quickly we can get the child off the breast. For some, weaning begins with formula, for others it's commercial baby food, usually made with left-over scrapings of products from the food industry.

My own children actually began weaning towards the end of their first year. Weaning isn't when your child stops breastfeeding completely, it's when you *start* replacing some breastfeeding sessions with other foods.

Our favourite weaning foods were strawberries, apple sucked on through organic muslin (which had been tied in a knot around it), mashed bananas, pears, peaches ~ all very ripe and fresh. Our girls have always loved fruit; and now they're completely weaned, they have no problem consuming 'five a day'.

They have never tasted commercial baby food. When they moved from fruits, raw and steamed vegetables, they began eating the same foods as Paul and I, such as lentil and vegetable hotpot, basmati rice, pinhead oatmeal. Their diet has always been rich and varied. They love food, and thrive on a high-raw, plant-based, wholefood diet. There are many ways to wean, but could it be that the only way which truly honours the child's needs is when they choose when and how, rather than having it imposed on them?

I believe it's important to think of breast milk as the only food for the first year of life. Consider the second year as a time for 'tasting' other foods. Every time you offer your baby a food, quietly ask yourself, "is it worth replacing breast milk with this?" If you ask yourself this consciously, rather than thinking or feeling pressured by "I need to introduce solids", you'll approach the transition from breast to other foods holistically, in a way which meets your baby's needs, rather than cultural expectations.

Enzymes

One of the big differences between breastfed and bottle-fed babies is in their approach to foods in childhood, and indeed in adulthood. Breastfed babies seem to have an in-built appreciation of natural, uncooked fruit, vegetables, seeds and nuts during and after weaning. This is because breast milk is enzyme-rich. (Fake milk has **no** enzymes.)

Enzymes are an unseen 'life force' within foods which contribute to our well-being, and aid digestion.

The Drinks Are On Me

Children who don't breastfeed in infancy have to deal with this deficiency of enzymes; and we see the consequences of this in the different rate of illness between bottle-fed and breastfed babies. The digestive patterns are vastly different in these two ways of feeding babies. The cultural addiction to junk foods is another example of the long-term impact of bottle-feeding fake milk.

Going back to work

Women often cite going back to work as a reason to wean. It need not be. You can breastfeed mornings and nights. You can breastfeed longer at weekends, or whenever you're off work. If women are clever enough, and creative enough, to make, birth and breastfeed a baby, then managing the art of work *and* mothering is not impossible. It's a choice. Choosing to continue the breastfeeding relationship will also provide comfort for your child when you reunite. We too easily underestimate and invalidate the *huge* emotional and psychological impact of a mother's absence. Many women say they go back to work so they don't get bored. Stay-at-home mothering doesn't *have* to be boring. Why not use it as a time for reflection, a place of self-discovery? We all have the need to be creative and express ourselves, there's no denying that. However, we can easily find ways to do so without separating ourselves from our children while they're young.

Night weaning of toddlers

It's highly likely that your child will want to breastfeed often through the night. And why wouldn't they? It's such lovely food for them, and they get to snuggle up with mamma in peace. The mistake some people make is comparing their breastfed, frequent-waking baby with the 'perfect' baby on artificial milk ~ who sleeps through the night without so much as a baby-sized snore. That baby is sleeping not because she's inherently 'good', and wishing to be kind to her parents ~ or, necessarily, content - but because artificial milk takes a heavy toll on the digestive system. When all the baby's energy goes into breaking the curds down and dealing with an enzyme-empty product, she has very little choice but to sleep. Her tiny body is exhausted. And bottle-feeding is no *guarantee* that baby will sleep through the night, so don't see it as an easy option. Of course, if you're completely exhausted, you will see your baby's night-time waking as a 'problem'.

Some simple ways to reduce night-time breastfeeding for an *older* baby/ toddler include allowing your child to breastfeed a lot more in the day time. Make sure your child isn't deprived of your touch; as far as possible carry her in a sling. Let the feed just before bedtime be a big one. Talk to your toddler in the night and say "breast milk in the morning". I used to say, "yes, you can have some breast milk when the sun wakes up." Some mothers have the baby sleep next to the dad, so the milk can't be smelt (and dreamt about!). Do this though, after your toddler has had a large feed, just prior to sleep.

The Drinks Are On Me

Learn to rub the baby's back, and change his position when he wakes, and see if this makes a difference.

As parents, it's tempting to always want to 'change things' with the baby if aspects of parenting are challenging. It's far healthier to change *our* life-style choices and expectations first. Then, we can look at what, perhaps, needs changing with the baby.

An important fact: your child won't do this forever.

Psychological well-being

Our brains are designed to develop at a certain rate, and each cell of our being has biological expectations. If the expectations for neuro-biological fulfilment are not met during the sequential development of brain growth, either because of parental negligence or ignorance, the synapses in the brain will simply fail to 'connect'. The connections shape us as adults. They determine how we'll relate to other human beings. Will we be intimate, trusting and loving? Or will we go through life feeling that nobody cares? Every affirmation of love by a parent ~ through breastfeeding, skin and eye contact and co-sleeping, meets a *neuro-biological* need. The blueprint of conscious, attachment parenting is vital to the long-term future of our children. If we miss nature's cues, there's no catching up at a later date.

One of the reasons cited by the vast majority of people for early weaning, is 'so that the child won't be dependent on the mother'. This is such unfortunate information to perpetuate, because breastfeeding is the ultimate way of offering psychological advantages to our children. And for the mother, it brings a natural and easy way to bond with her baby. The idea of a mother being a protective Mother Bear is more easily seen in those women who breastfeed. The hormones involved in breastfeeding bring up this healthy response, which is why our species has managed to survive for so long! The feel-good hormone, oxytocin, is vital for surviving. This is what creates the bonds which hold loving families together for generations.

We too easily
underestimate and invalidate
the huge
emotional and psychological impact
of a mother's absence.

The Drinks Are On Me

The psychological benefits our babies and children experience by being in their mother's arms and breastfeeding, are enhanced through skin and eye contact. It's well known in scientific circles that the bonds of attachment are built through this day-to-day give-and-take between mother and child. The baby learns to trust. Suckling from our mother makes us feel secure. The irony for humanity is that many people are now searching for spiritual insights and peak experiences. A breastfed baby has this every time she breastfeeds.

Neuro-biologists report changes in the human body when a baby is gazing into her mother's eyes while breastfeeding. As a natural mother, we sleep and carry our babies at all times, unless the baby wants to get down ~ which usually happens at around six months of age. We don't leave our infant alone, or baby-sat by a monitor, cctv, or left in a cot, pram or car seat.

Research shows that adults who were breastfed beyond the first year felt more comfortable with their body, and expressing body contact, than adults who were bottle-fed[27]. It is, understandably, very difficult for a bottle-feeding mother to hear, but the truth is that the love expressed through breastfeeding can't be replicated with a bottle, no matter how well intentioned the mother.

Actions speak louder than words. A baby needs to 'feel' your love, through eye contact, skin to skin touch, your heart beat, your presence and through the love contained *within* breast milk. Research into babies in orphanages found that babies who are not held at all, die. Regardless of how well-fed they are, or how excellent the hygiene, babies *need touch*[28]. In New York, during the early 1900s, many untouched babies died. Humans are a *continuous contact* species. It's vital to our bio-psycho-spiritual health and well-being. Every cell in our body craves this desire to be touched, and a baby needs this around the clock. So, the next time you hear someone say that breastfeeding makes a baby dependent, just smile, and agree. Yes, it *does* make a baby dependent, but not forever. The baby relies on her parent 100% to make sure she doesn't *die* from lack of touch.

It's a sad world we live in where we believe we can find the needs for human health in a factory, and for this to be the cultural norm. (Normal, in this case, doesn't mean natural). If our own lives weren't touched by breastfeeding in infancy, then it's easy to dismiss how important and vital it is for our own children. We rely on information and support from doctors and health visitors, and yet, they too may not have experienced mother love in the form of skin-to-skin, eye contact and other benefits which come from breastfeeding.

Have you ever wondered why some newspapers carry what have become known as page 3 models? These are topless women, usually with big breasts. Men seek out the breast in sexual ways to try and make up for their deprivation as infants and children. So, while they need the visual stimulus of topless models, they also require ways and means of stimulating the sucking experience.

Fingers, thumbs, sucking through a straw, cigarettes or cigars, sucking on a bottle, and talking non-stop. When the sucking need is met adequately at mother's breast, there's absolutely no need to utilise these self-soothing devices as an adult.

We have an epidemic of co-dependent adults in our culture. These are people who live their lives through others, rather than acknowledging their own true needs and desires. They have no real 'sense of self'. That is, they are *dependent* on someone else, emotionally, mentally or physically, to take care of them. It's tragic, but many, many people put up with all sorts of abuse, in order to keep someone's 'love'. This can be directly related to being deprived of the breast, or having breastfeeding end abruptly at an age when reasoning and logical thinking hasn't developed. We then search out someone to *take care of us* because our mother didn't.

"I'm NEVER going to wean!"
Eliza, at 5 years and 13 days.

Eliza began weaning near the end of her first year, with foods like avocado, strawberries and other soft, raw fruits.

How odd, that when she was less than *five months old*, the Plunket nurse (health care worker, New Zealand) wrote in her baby health book that Eliza was a "beautiful, happy-natured baby girl, exclusively breastfed, progressing well." She weighed 10.52 kg, had clear skin, mouth, eyes, and was an obviously healthy, thriving baby. She wrote *"introduce solids"*!!! What? At 5½ months she had two teeth. Common sense would tell you that a baby can't eat anything with just two teeth! Yet so many maternal health workers around the world give out just that sort of advice, and the tragedy is that most mothers unquestioningly follow such false information without giving it a second thought. As my friend Emma says, "we don't just give our babies food because they're interested in what we're eating. Our four year old is interested in watching us drive the car, but we wouldn't give him the keys and say 'drive'."

When Eliza was five or six years old, the amount of times she breastfed dropped enormously. She was well out of the needy-toddler stage, and busy with life. For whatever reason though, she enjoyed breastfeeding, and didn't seem to think of saying goodbye. Clearly, at a cellular level, her body knew breast milk was important for her brain. By the age of seven, she breastfed every few days, and sometimes only once every few weeks. People often assume older children breastfeed all the time. While toddler-hood is often a very intense time, usually by the age of three or so, children are less needy. I never asked her if she wanted to breastfeed. The choice always came from her ~ my attitude being very much along the lines of *'don't offer, don't refuse'*. The complete end of breastfeeding wasn't something that we ever discussed. Had it not been for the aforementioned tv documentary, Eliza's breastfeeding journey would have ended like Bethany's, quietly and without fuss.

Bethany had gone through a similar process when she was about six, and finally said goodbye around her seventh birthday, when she asked for 'one last feed'. Sometimes it's better not to know when the last breastfeed will be, because we risk giving it too much importance. Like the fading away of beautiful music, the memory is something you keep in your heart forever.

Breastfeeding beyond infancy ~ stepping past cultural taboos

Many breastfeeding organisations, as well as the World Health Organisation, recommend breastfeeding beyond infancy. The American Academy of Pediatrics (AAP) states that to breastfeed for less than two years *increases* a child's risk of disease. Yet despite all this high praise for continuing breastfeeding, we still see very little evidence of western women feeding children aged two and over. Given that less than 20 percent of mums in the UK feed past the six month mark, a toddler on the breast is a highly unlikely scenario.

It isn't surprising that women choose not to breastfeed after the first year or so, when our culture has such a bias against, and ignorance towards, breastfeeding. For many people it has a sense of being too primal, not suited to a civilised society. Others consider it to be in the realms of incest! The popularity of the page three breast photo in the UK's major tabloid papers, suggests that many people regard breasts as being sexual objects. In the face of such values, or lack thereof, it's a rare woman who will follow her intuition and buck the trend.

In the UK, the government has not issued any upper age limit for a child to stop breastfeeding. And yet the whole focus of the government towards family life is to make children as independent of their parents as possible ~ through early nursery care, incentives for early day care, etc. Studies have shown that children who have enjoyed full-term breastfeeding, contrary to popular belief, do not end up clingy, dependent and unable to function away from mother's skirt. That a child is dependent on her mother during the early years, rather than on a teddy bear, dummy or bottle, should be seen in a positive light.

Many people dismiss full-term breastfeeding because of their unfounded fears that the child will never wean. This is physically impossible, because the child loses the sucking reflex in their own time. And, as already stated, your body will make age-appropriate milk for your child and so she'll always benefit from it while still breastfeeding. Many families have also found it has a positive impact on family life. Rather than it ruining a couple's sex-life, as many people fear, the nurturing of a child's needs naturally, allows a deeper sense of intimacy to develop between the couple. They learn to respect the ebb and flow of hormones and feelings. Respect becomes the cornerstone of their relationship.

It's almost inevitable, on your breastfeeding journey, that someone will think they know better than you about when your child should wean. As far as possible, avoid taking the bait.

Ask the person if they'd genuinely like to know why you're still breast-feeding; and perhaps you could ask whether it makes them feel uncomfortable, and why. Often these situations, while initially dispiriting, remind us how far we've come in our parenting style, and they affirm what our priorities are.

Childhood caries ~ an artificial disease

All other mammals exclusively breastfeed their babies, yet humans are the only ones whose children develop Early Childhood Caries [ECC]. This would suggest that breast milk does *not* cause the decay, other foods or drinks do. Research has indicated that some infant formulas cause tooth decay by dissolving tooth enamel[29].

It's easy to assume, when a child's tooth enamel is not perfect, that breastfeeding must be the cause. This completely overlooks things such as heredity, and issues during gestation, such as the mother being ill with a virus, or being malnourished or stressed. Sometimes antibiotics taken in pregnancy, or given to the baby at birth, impact on tooth health. Shock and grief during pregnancy have been associated with tooth damage, decay and crumbling or blackening of baby teeth[30]. Be comforted that the adult teeth will be normal.

Common sense shows that humanity's teeth would not have lasted through time if breast milk was indeed the cause, quite simply because our evolution as a species was based on full-term breastfeeding, day and night. It's only in our comparatively recent history, when diets have diverged from nature's original intention, that we've seen major tooth decay[31]. Studies show that breast milk has anti-microbial properties and immunities which reduce bacteria. Fruit and vegetables, in their raw unprocessed state ~ such as strawberries, carrots, raspberries and avocados ~ contain ingredients known to have cavity-preventing properties. Herbs, too, such as mint, cloves and thyme, contain these ingredients.

Formula has been proven to be cariogenic. Please don't wean your child off breast milk in the mistaken belief that it's causing caries. Drinking from a bottle, because it's different than from a breast, means milk pools around the teeth. Breast milk taken from the breast doesn't sit in the mouth, it's expressed into the baby's throat.

Starch and sugar are the biggest culprits, and parents should consider their impact on a child's teeth. Many people overlook the fact that bread, for instance, turns to sugar in the mouth (as does any grain product).

A study found evidence to show that sustained breastfeeding didn't, in itself, lead to dental problems, such as caries[32]. The risk factors were large amounts of sugar-rich foods and drinks, family history, exposure to fluoride, the maternal diet during pregnancy, pre-maturity, and deficient dental hygiene.

Formula has also been found to be contaminated with dangerous toxic metals, fungal toxins, insecticides, and solvents[22]. The water used to *prepare* the formula is often polluted, and can lead to diarrhoea and other serious diseases. Chemicals also leach from formula bottles and cans into the formula mix. In their attempts to mimic breast milk, some formula companies include oils from palm trees. However, studies have shown this can affect the correct bone development of children.

Media reports state formula being recalled from consumers for containing things such as glass, and contaminants such as salmonella[23].

Reducing toxins in utero and in breast milk

Eat a largely plant-based diet. If you must eat meat or dairy, make it organic. The lower we eat on the food chain, the less toxins we take in through our food. Ideally, grow your own food, eat wild-crafted foods, or buy organic.

Drink fresh water. Tap water may contain fluoride, and will certainly contain chlorine.

Avoid alcohol, caffeine and drugs.

Clear chemicals from your home. Use vinegar, lemon and baking powder for cleaning. Avoid toxic solvents.

Use your concerns about toxins in the environment to clean up your own act. Changing your lifestyle is one step closer to changing the world around you.

It's impossible to buy fake milk which is free from genetic modification, unless labelled organic.

Teats for bottles are toxic[24].

Consider the impact of the furnishings in your home, such as carpets, curtains and furniture. In an ideal world we'd look at this well before conception, rather than panicking about it when we're breastfeeding. Modern houses abound with chemicals, such as formaldehyde in cooking gas, and in some brands of dishwashing liquid.

Eco-Feminism

Parenting can wreak havoc on Mother Earth. Equally, it can leave barely a footprint. The choice is ours. One of the most obvious examples is the choice to breastfeed over bottle-feeding. All breast milk is supplied at source, with no need for bottles, sterilising equipment, heating or electricity. It's available at all times.

To keep up with the increasing demand for artificial milk, more forests are being cleared ~ approximately 10,000 square metres per cow[25]. Deforestation leads to soil erosion. This is one of the biggest causes of nutrient-deficient soil. The topsoil is removed and it is here that most of the nutrients exist. They are vital for healthy plant growth. Soya is grown in these deforested areas, to feed the cattle needed to make milk.

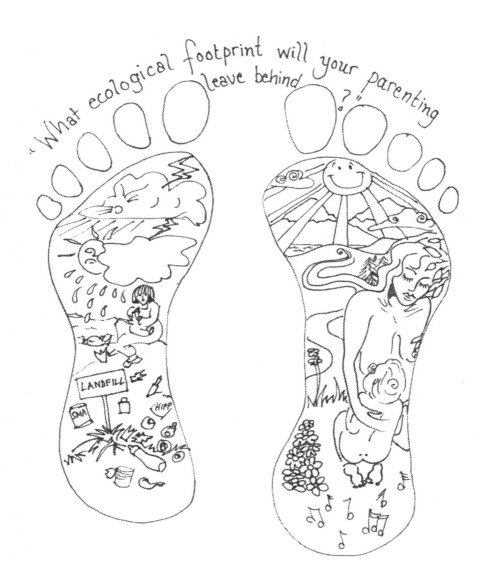

The Drinks Are On Me

A weaning party, anyone?

Katie Buchanan, producer of the channel four documentary Extraordinary Breastfeeding, no doubt with a keen eye on some good footage, or a twist in the Extraordinary Breastfeeding story, asked Eliza if she'd like a Weaning Party. It still makes me laugh; Eliza was enraged. Hands on hips, and with the full-force of a tidal wave, she disbelievingly asked, "A weaning party? A *weaning* party? *I don't want to wean!*"

Never mind. Anyway, who would we have invited? The Queen? I don't think she gives MBEs to seven year olds. (Mourning the Breastfeeding Experience).

Some parents do offer weaning parties to their older children, to coincide with the child's conscious choice to finish breastfeeding. There are plenty of children who just decide that they've finished with it, and say matter-of-factly that they won't be asking any more. Whether or not their sucking reflex was losing its grip because of their non-interest, or it came from a place of increased emotional security, it's hard to know. Often it comes from outside pressure ~ friends, family or strangers. Clearly, the reasons will be different for each child.

It's absolutely vital that regardless of when a child or baby is weaned, a mother and father take into full consideration all the emotional and nutritional needs. They'll need to be met in other ways, though clearly it will be inferior to feeding at the breast. A mother returning to work is usually the catalyst for weaning, and yet this is the very time the child most needs the reassurance of breastfeeding. Children under the age of three have no concept of "mummy's coming back later".

Weaning can be very traumatic for a baby/child. Sadly, it's a psychological transition that's rarely respected in our quick-quick culture. We should look to our children's teeth as a very clear indicator of when to wean. They're still emerging after two years of age. Mother's milk is vital in building up the bones, which are increasing in density for the first five years. The WHO figure of breastfeeding into the second year and *beyond*, has been drawn from many fields: medical, biological, psychological and anthropological.

The current world-wide *average* age for weaning is four years old. This shows that when children are left to breastfeed naturally, they will do so for much longer than we see in the west. This average includes all the children who breastfeed for only a day or two, which means that many children around the world are breastfeeding for *much longer* than four years. Their actions speak louder than any theories put forward by child care experts.

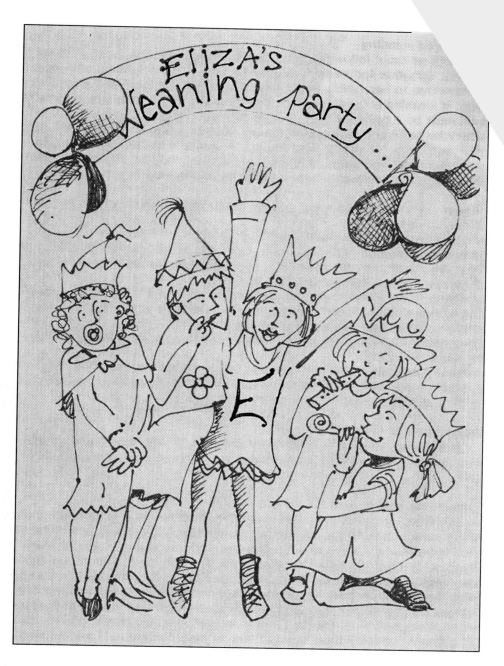

And what about weaning parties for children who suck on dummies, pens, fingers, thumbs, hair, lolly pops... Will anyone expect them to wean?

The Drinks Are On Me

' her baby's leads rather than other people's expec-
...ning programme should <u>always</u>, and in all ways,
needs. Gradually eliminate one feed every few
...ing place before the baby is nine months old, breast
...stituted by a nutritionally suitable milk. Give serious con-
...o this choice, as formula can never come remotely close to what
...wn body is capable of providing. Always remember your baby's im-
...nune system is immature, and no other food or drink has the capability of
developing it, or his brain, as beautifully and effectively as breast milk.

Unnecessary weaning advice usually comes about in response to the following circumstances:
Mastitis *[weaning is the worst thing to do!].*
Overwhelmed by mothering *[formula feeding is unlikely to change this].*
Teething *[most cultures breastfeed long after all the teeth are through. Breastfeeding is nature's analgaesic.]*
Mother or baby ill/hospitalised *[A sick baby needs the anti-infective properties of breast milk. A mother may get mastitis from abrupt weaning. A distressed mother and baby will compromise healing].*
Drugs *[most medicinal drugs are breastfeeding compatible. Substitutes can be found for others].*
Returning to work *[breastfeeding is easier for mother and child].*
Pregnancy *[does not hurt the baby in utero. Mother should keep up her nutrition, she might consider tandem nursing].*

Ways to wean
Mother-led weaning is often done abruptly, though some times gradually, partially or planned. The only *natural* way to wean, is when it is child-led.

Introducing foods
When beginning solids, always breastfeed **first** to keep up your milk supply. A hungry baby is less inclined to try new foods. A stable intake of calories is maintained by a balance of breast milk and solids. Introduce new foods on a spoon, as finger foods, cubed soft foods, berries or grated fruit and vegetables. In ancient times, mothers (and modern mothers in touch with their intuitive side) would chew their babies' food so it contained the mother's *digestive* enzymes. Consider doing this with your baby's food, as it will help digestion enormously. Don't necessarily expect your mother-in-law or strangers to understand though. Ripe *organic* bananas are a great first food, and so are avocados. Try to stick with raw foods at first, and avoid introducing grains until well into the third year.

If you're concerned about iron, offer baby some organic dried apricots which have been soaked well overnight. Blend to a purée. These are easy to digest. Children who are exclusively breastfed for at least seven months have iron stores for life, unlike those babies weaned at six months or earlier. The breastfeeding mother's diet should be rich in natural wholefoods and plenty of nutritious liquids. Drink to thirst. You know you're drinking enough if your urine is pale and odourless.

Common allergens

A baby may be allergic to the following foods (either through breast milk, or eaten directly): cow's milk; eggs; citrus; berries; saturated fats; salt; sugar; honey. Typical symptoms of a food allergy in a breastfed baby include: diarrhoea; irritable intestines; rash; hives; green watery stools; vomiting; wheezing; asthma; congestion; ear infection; fussiness; colic; red, itchy eyes and sore bottom.

If the allergy is mild, eliminate the suspected foods from your diet until the child is older. It can take two to three days or even up to a week to eliminate suspected food from your body. If severe, consult a breastfeeding specialist.

Child-led weaning

Child-chosen weaning situations tend to happen at about four or five years of age. It seems such a short space of time in terms of the human lifetime. To wean a child before this time is *premature* weaning. Biologically, a human child expects to breastfeed anywhere up to seven years. Beyond this age might then be called "extended breastfeeding". The benefits of child-led weaning/extended breastfeeding are numerous.

According to research, breastfed children are physically healthier[52]. Breast milk is nearly always accepted by an ill child when no other food or liquid is wanted. It also offers protection to an allergic child. But it's not just the child who benefits. It allows the mother to slow down and relax. It makes the job of comforting and nurturing a toddler easier. Mothers who breastfeed longer are at less risk of cancer. Exclusive breastfeeding can provide for natural child spacing.

When women once again listen to their intuitive voice, they'll know that although raising a child naturally takes an enormous amount of time and energy, it also brings a beautiful and irreplaceable, intimate connection. The children of such women won't form attachments to inanimate objects in the hope of getting their needs met. *Instead, they'll form healthy, life-long relationships, and most importantly, will not be afraid to love*[53].

Studies reveal a much lower divorce rate amongst people who received long-term breastfeeding as children[61].

The Drinks Are On Me

WHOLEFOODS *to introduce during the weaning years*

It helps to become familiar with the variety of wholefoods which exist, so that you have them readily at your fingertips when preparing meals for your family. In the UK, it takes the average woman four days to move food from her mouth out of her body. This clearly *isn't* healthy! In an adult, healthy bowels move 2 - 4 times a day ~ easily, and without strain, releasing food from the day before. Set up healthy habits for your weaning child so they'll stay with her for life. Avoid ready-made baby foods. They're deficient in vital digestive enzymes.

Fruits
Melons
Berries
Tropical fruits
Stone fruits
Citrus
Vine fruits
(Fruits can be fresh or dried, though dried should be a treat, not a staple. Fruit which has been tinned, bottled or frozen is not considered fresh).

Vegetables
All leafy greens
Salad vegetables (tomato, cucumber, peppers)
Root vegetables
Sea vegetables

Seeds
Sunflower
Pumpkin
Sesame
Poppy
Linseed (flax)
Hemp
(Seeds are best eaten when sprouted or soaked overnight).

Pulses
Lentils
Peas
Beans

Whole grains
Brown basmati rice
Quinoa
Pinhead oatmeal
Millet
Corn
Barley
Buckwheat
(Wheat is also a grain, but not suited to human digestion, so use it sparingly, rather than as a staple).

Nuts
Almonds
Hazelnuts
Macadamias
Cashew
Peanuts (really a legume)
Pecans
Brazils
Pine nuts
Pistachios
Walnuts

(Nuts should be eaten raw. For toddlers, you can homogenise nuts to make nut butters. You can also make wonderful sorbets, sauces and creams from fruit, for babies being introduced to solids. To make nut butters, you'll need a juicer with a 'blank' blade which is capable of homogenising.)

Herbs and spices ~ dried and fresh

Oils
Flaxseed
Hempseed
Olive
Coconut
Sesame
Olive, coconut and sesame oil are suitable for cooking.

Sweeteners
Agave syrup
Raw honey *(not for children under 12 months of age)*
Rice malt
Stevia

Drinks
Water!
Herb teas
Freshly made fruit and vegetable juices

Others
Apple cider vinegar
Tofu
Miso

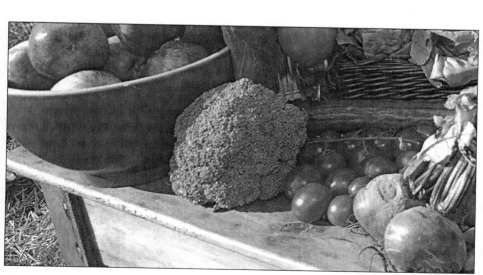

The Drinks Are On Me

When a baby dies

My mum remembers when she was a child and being asked to drink from her mother's breasts, which were full of milk after the death of a sibling. My grandmother Leiselotta's breasts were aching in more ways than one. Her body was desperate for relief from the all-consuming engorgement, and every cell in her body was mourning the loss of this infant. She lost three babies in infancy.

Doctors may offer drugs to dry up milk. This is unnecessary and certainly not the only option. Although the drying up of milk may bring relief, for some women it is like another 'death'.

The tragic circumstances in which some women find their breasts are full but their arms are empty, can make the passing of their baby as physically traumatic as it is emotionally, mentally and spiritually.

Although it's perfectly acceptable to allow the breasts to dry up on their own, through lack of demand, some women would rather not have leaky breasts as it's a further reminder of their loss. In this case, I recommend drinking sage tea. It's available in all good health stores, or, if you have it growing in your garden, infuse some in hot water, and drink several cups throughout the day for up to a week. You might prefer to sweeten it with a little honey or agave syrup. Sage tea, unlike prescribed drugs, has no harmful side effects when taken as directed. Even when lactation ends, some women have milk in their breasts for up to three years. Herbs such as sage help to diminish supply.

Some mothers, upon the death of their baby, have chosen to act as a wet nurse for mums who, for whatever reason, were unable to breast feed. Other mothers hand express their milk in the shower and let it wash away with the water. They use the privacy of the shower to cry away both their pain and their breast milk. Donating the milk to a milk bank for babies in NICU or SCBU, or specifically for a baby whose mother has died, has helped some mothers find a creative, and, literally, expressive way to deal with this painful and difficult time. Each mother has to do what intuitively feels right.

If you've lost your infant, you might like to create a garden where you can bury the body or ashes, and plant flowers or plants which blossom annually as a reminder of the child's birth/death. Some women choose to see their drops of breast milk as tears, and they trust their body to stop crying in its own time. They catch these tears and use this *living water* to nourish and give life to the plants. Families have found this very healing and therapeutic.

The death of a child is not something you get over, but something you learn to live with. No-one, not even another parent who's lost a child in similar circumstances, can, or should, tell you when to stop grieving. It's a uniquely personal experience. It's so important that you honour your grieving process, in your own way, no matter how long it takes.

Our hungry brain

Why we NEED human milk

There are many reasons why breastfed children are more intelligent than they would have been had they been formula-fed. One reason is that breastfed babies have more interaction with their parents ~ more holding, touching, more eye-contact. This is vital for correct neuro-biological development. Formula-fed babies are much more likely to be given a dummy to comfort them, and as a result, less oxygen will get to the baby's brain.

Another reason for higher intelligence is to do with the superior nutrients in breast milk ~ nutrients *specific* to brain growth. DHA, a fat in breast milk, is found in much greater quantities in the brains of breastfed babies. In order to help your child's brain development, it's important you include DHA in your diet too (see below). All this goodness will be received by your baby in the breast milk. Cholesterol, a scary word for adults, is actually important for babies, and vital in brain development. No surprise then, that breast milk has a lot of cholesterol.

The essential fats are so important for our baby, that even if our diet is lacking them, our breasts are capable of creating them 'on the go'. The natural sugar found in breast milk, lactose, gets broken down into galactose and glucose. The amount of lactose in a mamma's milk is proportionate to the level of intelligence of the species. Humans have much higher lactose than cows.

Although the human body can't make essential fatty acids, it does require them, as they're absolutely necessary for building the brain and supporting the nervous system. When we consume omega 3 and omega 6 fatty acids, our body converts them to Eicosapentaenoic Acid (EPA) and Docosahexaenoic Acid (DHA). As a result, our cell membranes are made more flexible, allowing both the releasing of toxins out of the body, and the taking in of nutrients.

Our body converts the omega oils into what are known as long-chain polyunsaturated fatty acids. Commonly referred to as omega 3, this fatty acid, otherwise known as *alpha linolenic acid*, becomes EPA and DHA. Fish is commonly recommended. However, all we have to do is consume the EPA and DHA through algae-based foods and we too can obtain the essential fats directly. Research from London's King's College found that algae is a far more potent source of Omega 3 DHA than fish oil[33]. During pregnancy, it's vital we eat foods rich in DHA, so our baby has the optimal chance of developing its nervous system and brain.

Linoleic acid, known commonly as omega 6, is required to balance female hormones, among other things. This is converted in our body to arachidonic acid (AA). In our culture there's a danger of consuming too much, as it's readily found in dairy and meat.

The Drinks Are On Me

Over-consumption of AA has been linked to cardiovascular and arthritic complaints ~ again, another reason to consume plant-based omega 6. Some people have difficulty converting EFAs because of a health condition, such as an atopic allergy (eczema, hay fever and asthma) and diabetes. It is recommended they purchase an EPA/DHA algae supplement.

Reasons not to obtain your essential fatty acids from oily fish:
*Ethical sources exist in the plant world.
*Toxicity (dioxins, mercury, PCPs) found in fish.
*Commercially farmed fish require antibiotics etc., because of the unnatural conditions in which they live, and the processed foods which they are forced to eat. There's no evidence to show they're able to convert omega oils in this environment from the foods they eat.

Lifestyle changes to increase your absorption of essential fatty acids
Your ability to convert EFAs to EPA and DHA is affected by smoking, alcohol, viral infections such as herpes, animal fats and trans fats in processed foods, stress, excess vitamin A, caffeine (coffee, coke, chocolate, tea, some painkillers) and excess copper. Include in your meals, each day, the oils from nuts and seeds, as well as eating them whole. Try having spirulina smoothies, chorella, E3 Live, or Nature's Living Superfood every other day.

To be able to convert EPAs, ensure your diet is rich in vitamins B3 and B6, zinc, biotin, vitamin C, calcium and magnesium. Omega 3 and omega 6 oils need to be balanced. Commonly, people have far too much omega 6, because sunflower oil is used in abundance in processed foods. Have about 1 part of omega 3 to 3 parts of omega 6. If you need oils for cooking, the best two are coconut oil and cold-pressed olive oil. All oils should be kept cold, in dark glass containers.

Sources of omega 6 oil (Linoleic Acid)
Vegetables; fruits; nuts; grains; seeds
Oils made from safflower; sunflower; corn; soya; evening primrose; pumpkin; wheatgerm

Sources of omega 3 oil (Alpha-Linolenic Acid)
(Please note - fish is not the only source of omega 3 acids. Flaxseed oil contains twice as much as is found in fish oil!).
Flaxseeds (linseeds); mustard seeds; green leafy vegetables; grains; spirulina; pumpkin seeds; soya beans; walnuts
Oils made from linseeds (flaxseeds), rapeseeds (canola), soya beans and walnuts.

All you need is love (love, love...)

Studies of adults with a history of violence, depression, suicidal tendencies and criminal acts show that they all have in common a reduced level of serotonin in their bodies[34]. This is a chemical in the brain which is reduced when the *affectionate* loving and bonding between mother and child aren't adequate. Colostrum, the first milk our body produces, contains tryptophan, an *essential* ingredient for developing serotonin. This *isn't* in artificial milk.

Throughout our mammalian history we've had these two aspects, the physiological component of breastfeeding, and the psychological benefits of *mother love* and attention from continuous contact, supporting each other in order to help the babies of our species grow their brains and bodies optimally.

Our whole cultural way of modern parenting ~ separating mother and child at birth for tests etc. ~ and encouraging the use of formula milk, has led to a devastating impact on humanity. This is completely opposed to nature's plan for us as human beings. Add to all this the vast number of babies not *ever* being breastfed, and therefore also not benefiting from oxytocin (the love hormone) ~ another neuro-chemical process of the brain absolutely necessary for helping the mother-child bond ~ then how can we possibly be surprised at such high incidences of drug and alcohol abuse, dysfunctional behaviour, depression and violence?

A recent study into the differences between children raised on formula and those who were breastfed, concluded that children who didn't receive breast milk were significantly more likely to have an autistic disorder[35].

If only we could change our parenting practices and have **all** children breastfed and receiving nurturing and nourishment, nature's way, we could transform the world into a more peaceful place.

Breastfeeding and memory

Dopamine is a powerful regulator, and it integrates aspects of brain function. It contributes to how we adapt to behaviour. It's part of a complex neural network in our mid-brain, commonly known as the 'reward pathway'. It prompts good feelings in response to certain behaviours, such as when it is produced breastfeeding. This promotes early bonding and specifically reduces stress. The pleasurable aspect of breastfeeding, an increase in alertness and the ability to develop memory, are the result of opoids (pleasure hormones) and oxytocin (love hormone).

The Drinks Are On Me

Full-term breastfeeding

Given that throughout most of history, humans have breastfed their babies full-term (at least six or seven years of age), our recent blip of sixty or so years experimenting with substitutes, and premature weaning, will not have 'yet' changed our genetic structure. However, if we don't reclaim breastfeeding, the consequences will be absolutely dire. The symptoms of not breastfeeding are already manifesting in an assortment of ways, and the price is high.

The needs of a young child are many. First and foremost, society looks to the physical needs. Wrongly, we assume that breast milk can be adequately replaced with other milks, or foods, at the most tender age. Physically, **breast** milk is needed to build the brain. Breastfeeding itself is needed emotionally, psychologically and spiritually. Breastfeeding beyond six months or so is often called *extended* breastfeeding. But language can be very directive, and equally, it can be downright misleading. Extended, in this case, suggests that the practice involves doing something 'beyond' a certain time, whereas **full-term** breastfeeding is an expression which accurately describes the time involved in a child breastfeeding till her needs are met.

But when is a child too old to breastfeed? Funnily enough, for all the squeamishness exhibited by the Great British Public when my daughter Bethany declared on national tv that she wanted to breastfeed for her 9th birthday present, the UK government doesn't have any law stating the maximum age a child can breastfeed. So, where do we look for ideas on what is the 'right' age to finish the breastfeeding relationship?

Well, at the risk of stating the obvious, the first place we should look is to the children themselves. Clearly though, we can't look to the vast majority of kids in our western culture, because they're drinking cow's milk from as early as day one. It's important to recognise the huge shock for a newborn in not getting their needs met by being denied breastfeeding. Add to this, modern birth practices and being born into an alien environment after utero, and we see just how compromised many western babies are right from the beginning of life.

In many countries, breastfeeding *does* continue well into childhood, two to three years and longer. For example, by about two years of age, at least a third of the children in sub-Saharan Africa are still breastfeeding.

According to a World Health Organisation report, campaigns to encourage breastfeeding for two years were successful in increasing rates in developing countries[36]. Of course, now, with the Baby-Friendly Initiatives to promote breastfeeding in place in many hospitals around the world, most of the focus is on getting babies to breastfeed exclusively for the first few months, so no thought is given to older children breastfeeding.

In rural China, a study on <u>exclusive</u> breastfeeding for up to 12 months (i.e. no other foods or drinks are consumed), combined with further breastfeeding, resulted in good growth and nutritional status[37]. Such a study could never be carried out in the UK or Australia, the USA/Canada or New Zealand, because so few children are breastfed beyond six months. In five out of seven Asian countries studied, 50% or more were still being breastfed at two years; in Bolivia, Peru and Guatemala, 40% of children; and in Indonesia 63% of children are still breastfed at this age[38]. It would be wrong to assume that breastfeeding is a Third World activity simply because they don't have the resources to nourish their children in any other way. Breastfeeding is an area where developing nations are in advance of western countries. Although the west may have advantages in terms of resources for nutrition after breastfeeding, those advantages are being built on the flimsy foundations of infant formula.

A study found that child under-nutrition had no association with prolonged breastfeeding, only with poverty and illiteracy[39].

Anthropological evidence shows that humans have evolved to breastfeed for several years. Duration of breastfeeding is affected by all aspects of our culture. Biologically and historically, in most cultures, sustained breastfeeding is normal. Anthropologist Katherine Dettwyler asked, in 1995, what the natural age of weaning would be if we were free from cultural beliefs. She looked at the age of weaning in other large mammals, particularly the primates that are closest to humans, and estimated the natural age of weaning to be between two and a half to seven years of age.

The signs for weaning in large mammals and primates include quadrupling of birth weight, attainment of one-third adult weight, adult body size, gestation length, and dental eruption. In humans, quadrupling of birth weight occurs at around 27 months for males and around 30 months for females.

Anthropologists who compared the weaning ages of humans to primates concluded it would be natural to wean half way to sexual maturity, which is about seven in humans. It's well known that the immune system of a baby is immature and doesn't develop fully until about seven years of age. Common sense would suggest that antibodies in the mother's milk would be an ally to supporting immune function. Studies of monkeys and apes have shown weaning to occur about the time of getting their first permanent molars. In humans this is about six years of age. Another study showed that primates weaned at about 1/3 of adult weight. In humans this could be about six to seven years of age.

Our culture does not value breastfeeding. Combine that with a predominantly nuclear family-based society, and it's obvious that mothers who wish to breastfeed longer than the norm will have to seek out support. All of these studies lead us to the conclusion that it's **biologically** natural to breastfeed up to about seven years of age, with the earliest weaning happening at about two and a half.

The Drinks Are On Me

All around the world, in cultures where it's 'normal' to allow children to breastfeed as long as they want, they'll tend to wean *from* about four years of age. They do so without any distress. The immune system of a child who breastfeeds full-term is strengthened greatly by breast milk. Such children are ill less often than children fed on artificial milk. In 1993, children who'd been breastfed for up to two years were part of a study which showed higher IQ and school grades, in relation to longer breastfeeding[40]. Another study, showed the cognitive ability of seven and eight year old children was higher within those who'd been breastfed for eight months or more[41]. The mother's memory of breastfeeding was cross-referenced with hospital and child-health record books.

Long-term breastfeeding lessens the incidence of being overweight and obese later in life[42]. Another study found that toddlers who breastfed for longer than 12 months tended to have relaxed mothers who were less likely to dictate the way their toddler consumed food and drink. These children often had a much more varied diet[43]. In 1999, a study done on the Darling Downs, Queensland, Australia, showed that when children were still partially breastfed at 12 months, they were given significantly less inappropriate foods and drinks ~ such as cordial, creamy cow's milk, sugary drinks, soya formula[44]

A study by the WHO suggests that just half a litre of breast milk a day provides almost half the daily allowance of Vitamin A, almost all Vitamin C and about 1/3 of the protein and energy requirements that a child needs in its second year of life[45].

The authors of a 1999 study followed infants who were born before their due date. They found that the greater the amount of breast milk received, the greater their bone mineralization. They concluded that extended breastfeeding was optimal for bone mineral acquisition[46].

It has been shown that long-term breastfeeding children were more able to form attachments to others, and to become more independent than their bottle-fed peers[47]. In adolescence, these teenagers considered that their mothers weren't over-protective, but more caring[48]. There are many benefits for the mother, such as reduced risk of osteoporosis, breast cancer, anaemia; and the ability to shed postpartum weight. Cessation of menstrual periods can provide natural contraception during exclusive breastfeeding. Women who've breastfed for longer than a total of six years show a significantly reduced risk of breast cancer[49]. This study was done in China and Japan. Again, it would be more difficult to do such a study in the west, because of our cultural bias against breastfeeding full-term.

What is it like to breastfeed an older child?

In many ways it isn't a lot different to breastfeeding a newborn or toddler, in that it provides comfort, reassurance, nutrition and love. A toddler manages to learn breastfeeding gymnastics, and finds all sorts of positions to breastfeed in ~ some funny, and some downright annoying.

Little boys like to use breast milk to top up their toy tractor. Apparently it makes them run better than diesel! Girls like to feed their dolls with breast milk. They *know!*

Usually, by the age of four or five, the monkey-like antics have settled down, and the child is more than happy to have a peaceful breastfeeding session, either on the sofa next to you, or lying down in bed. Sometimes it's once a day, other times days or even weeks may go by. It certainly doesn't tend to be intense like the early years of breastfeeding. For me, not breast-feeding in public beyond the age of about four or five was one aspect which was significantly different from the early years. This wasn't to do with any hang-ups I had, but out of respect for the general public. At this age, a child is very understanding about breastfeeding only happening in private.

The main difference is clearly the size of the child, in that they don't just tuck up into your lap the way a baby does. And it's this reason, proba-bly more than any other, that has most people balking at the idea of sus-tained breastfeeding. In our culture, we associate breastfeeding with a tiny baby who doesn't take up much space. If we had more visual references to full-term breastfeeding, we'd start to see it as normal.

The film crew who made Extraordinary Breastfeeding is a good case in point; they got so used to the sight of toddlers and older children breast-feeding, that they started to find it as normal as the sight of a newborn at the breast. It really is just about a person's frame of reference. There was a time in my life when I found the sight of an older child breastfeeding to be odd. All of us are capable of stretching and expanding our belief systems.

Children who can talk about their breastfeeding experiences tend to do so eloquently, with real appreciation and passion. At some point this must provide a key to changing the mass consciousness. After all, if full-term breastfeeding is so wrong, then surely our children would be the first to tell us!

When I was a guest on a hideous tv 'chat' show, one member of the audi-ence suggested that children aren't 'in their right mind', so they don't know it's "wrong to breastfeed". Sigh. Babies and children who breastfeed are in touch with the Source of all life. They are far more in their *right mind* than most adults will ever be.

Contrary to popular belief, full-term breastfeeding isn't a selfish act on the mother's part. It isn't about her 'holding on to her children'. To con-sciously choose full-term breastfeeding is a selfless act, and to enjoy it fully we need to prioritise mothering. *You can't force a baby or child to breast-feed.* The mother can not make a child feed at the breast. It has to come willingly. That children will breastfeed for years on end is indicative of how pleasurable it is; and, as adults, we can learn a lot by honouring our chil-dren's needs.   For example, a recent UK study, which set out to prove co-sleeping with babies was harmful, found the complete opposite! Their con-clusions showed that by sleeping with our child for at least **five** years, their physical, emotional and psychological well-being were greatly enhanced[50].

The Drinks Are On Me

Non-nutritive sucking

Ultrasound scans show some babies suck their thumbs in utero. Once born, however, children suck their thumb as a form of self-soothing. Sometimes it begins in order to satisfy physical discomfort, such as teething or ear ache. It's symptomatic of a baby/child using it to satisfy an unmet need. Breastfeeding advocates put so much focus on the nutrients in breast milk and how they build up the immune system, that non-nutritive sucking is routinely overlooked, and usually misunderstood.

Many mothers feed their baby/child from both breasts in one sitting, and the session finishes when the child's tummy is full. This is unique in western culture, even among women who practise attachment parenting. Putting breastfeeding in the category of food misses out half the picture. Breast-feeding is an important bonding time. *Non-nutritive sucking* is a misnomer. Our children receive abundant nutrition and sustenance from sucking on an 'empty' breast. It allows the child to study your face. This aspect of bonding is vital for a healthy sense of well-being. Our child, by engaging in so-called *non-nutritive sucking*, isn't wasting our time, or as some people suggest, just 'using us as a dummy'. He's developing non-verbal communication, learning to trust, and receiving the hormone oxytocin (the love hormone).

Unfortunately, our society doesn't recognise the necessity of sucking, despite the deprivation of it manifesting all around us in adults and children. It's a huge need for *every* human being. As breastfeeding mothers, we can put our baby back on the 'empty' breast and allow him to keep suckling.

Every child is different and some will need to suckle more than others. The nurturing which occurs in the breastfeeding relationship allows our children to flourish. Through *non-nutritive sucking* we offer company, security, bonding and the release of positive hormones.

Medicine cabinet

According to ancient mythology, when the Greek Goddess Hera had orgasms, her breast milk squirted across the heavens ~ hence, our Milky Way, the Galaxy from the Great Galactagogue.

Poor old Hera, I know what she went through! My milk was always spraying, landing on our ceiling, wardrobe doors, the dashboard in the car. That's not to say I was having orgasms everywhere, but hormones and mother's let-down response meant that, more often than not, just *thinking* about my baby caused my breasts to leak milk. Your breast milk is a magical medicine cabinet, with everything you need to keep your baby healthy.

Breast milk is sterile, as well as anti-bacterial. It can be used topically for blisters and cold sores. The most common use by far is for conjunctivitis. Simply squirt directly from your breast into the corner of your baby's eyes. Do this several times a day. It's perfect for sore and cracked nipples, but *only* if you don't have thrush. Yeast loves to grow in breast milk. After rubbing milk into your nipples, allow them to air dry. Breast milk is wonderful for all sorts of cuts, scratches and scrapes. Clean the wound with your breast milk and then allow it to air dry. For ear infections, squirt into the sore ear. It's also helpful for a stuffed nose; use it in place of the normally recommended salt solution. Breast milk is wonderfully soothing for skin, and can be used for nappy rash, eczema and acne. Again, as with wounds, clean first with breast milk, then allow to air dry. Insect bites, such as those from ants and mosquitoes, respond well to breast milk. It alleviates itching. Apply to sunburn and fire burns. Its healing properties are nothing short of miraculous, and mothers have been using it in myriad ways down the ages.

There's a record of breast milk being used in the 16th century BC to heal a variety of things, such as eczema, cataracts, burns and scalding. Swedish doctors have discovered breast milk to be a highly effective treatment for warts. 80% of patients who used a breast milk lotion noticed lasting effects. The key ingredient was Alphalactalbumin (as hard to say as it is to write!). You can put breast milk directly onto the wart, without having to buy the lotion.

HERBS to avoid if breastfeeding

Black walnut, periwinkle sorrel, chickweed, lemon balm, spearmint, thyme, peppermint, yarrow, sage, parsley, wormwood, elecampane, ginseng, angelica root, rhubarb, kava kava, buckthorn, uva ursi, star anise, coltsfoot. These herbs impact on the supply of breast milk and may cause it to stop altogether. Some of them upset the baby's tummy.

Women who believe they can't breastfeed

One of the most common reasons for women not breastfeeding is the mistaken belief that they have insufficient milk. Medically, this situation has become known as "insufficient milk syndrome". It's unique to countries where artificial milk is readily available.

The 'feeling' of insufficient milk is a direct result of a lack of nipple stimulation by the baby. We cannot correct this by offering a baby formula milk. It's in the interests of fake milk companies to promote the 'idea' of insufficient milk syndrome. The worst advice we can give a woman who worries she has low milk, is to tell her to give her baby formula!

The most important thing we bring to the decision of breastfeeding is our attitude to embrace it fully, both for our self and our child. Ultimately, it's about taking responsibility, not only for our own well-being and health, but that of our child and future generations.

For all the wonders and benefits of our modern world, when it comes to how we feed our children, we've got too many options available. If there was no choice but to breastfeed, from the breast, I doubt we'd hear a peep regarding insufficient milk syndrome. A mother would move heaven and earth to make sure her milk came through.

The greatest support we can give others is compassion. It's easy to confuse that with supporting the myth of insufficient milk syndrome. By perpetuating the myth that some women 'don't make breast milk', we let all women, and babies, down. I know there'll be women reading this who either feel they couldn't breastfeed, or can vouch for someone else who 'couldn't feed'.

Let's debunk this once and for all. If you've got breasts which haven't been damaged by surgery, and you've birthed your baby, you *can* breastfeed. This myth of 'not being able to make milk' is *never* seen in indigenous cultures.

We're mammals. Our bodies are designed to make milk. What would make someone think they've got a faulty model? If you couldn't breastfeed, it was because you didn't have the *right support* (emotional, physical, psychological and spiritual) to show you how ~ to teach you the law of *supply and demand*, and advise on how to allow your body to 'let down'.

Your mind is more powerful than anything on the planet. Use it to help establish breastfeeding. Your body can do this. Don't allow anyone to convince you otherwise.

If you need help right now with your milk supply:
Think milk. Visualise your breasts filling with milk, and not baby.
Avoid bottles and pacifiers and formula.
Check position and latch-on. *If you don't know what a correct latch looks like get advice from an experienced breastfeeding mother. You can always contact La Leche League or your nearest breastfeeding support group.*
Nurse frequently.
Allow plenty of time at each feed so baby gets hindmilk.
Look after yourself.
Make breastfeeding a priority, and a pleasant experience.
Make a nurturing breastfeeding environment for you and your baby.
Talk to your baby often.
Touch her.
Feed her as much as she desires.
Limit your activities to just nursing your baby.

If you feel your milk is low, consider the following factors:
If you answer yes to any of these, you should tell your lactation consultant or other breastfeeding expert, as these can impact milk supply.
Did you sustain injuries during birth?
Were you given morphine during birth?
Did all of the placenta come out?
Are you taking any medications?
Are you on a contraceptive pill?
Is your baby ill?

Safe herbs to increase milk supply:
Fennel, fenugreek and caraway seeds. Stew them in a tea, or sprout for use in salads. Goat's rue can increase milk by up to 50%. They can all be bought in health stories.

Other tinctures/teas to consider:
Borage; raspberry leaves; blessed thistle; cinnamon; false unicorn root; garlic; dill nettles; saw palmetto; chaste tree

Essential oil
Essential oil of jasmine is very effective against severe depression and should be considered if you've had a medically managed/interfered with birth. It's also beneficial for bringing milk down. Blend with grape or almond oil and ask someone to give you a massage, or use in an oil burner.

Maintain a diet rich in seeds, nuts and fresh fruits. Eat vegetables raw. Include alfalfa sprouts, carrots and watercress.

The Drinks Are On Me

Flower essences can increase your milk supply

There are so many helpful flower essences that can support a nursing mother, that it's worth looking into as an aid to opening the heart chakra ~ a requirement for breastfeeding. (See chapter Finding our heart centre).

Nui (coconut) ~ stimulates the natural breastfeeding instinct in mothers.
Pear flower essence ~ a maternal essence helpful for those who are worried. Helps with breastfeeding.
Impatiens ~ to learn confidence with one's own body, and allowing closeness between mother and baby. Strengthens self-esteem.
St John's Wort ~ for a tendency to confusion and lack of self confidence, gives trust in the future and a belief in the good ending of all things. Can help with communication problems in a partnership.
Mariposa lily ~ to bring balance to women who are alienated from mothering, or have feelings of childhood abandonment/abuse. *All of these essences are available through the International Flower Essence Repertoire.*

The suck of a baby is different to manual and electronic breast pumping. Don't use these as a guide to your milk supply, instead, look to your baby's nappies. There should be six to eight really wet nappies a day. Only use a pump when you're unable to be with your baby, or trying to induce lactation. If your baby can feed directly from your breast, <u>always</u> choose this over pumping. To increase our milk supply we need to promote the hormone prolactin. This is *always* stimulated by a baby feeding on your breast. Keep feeding your baby. Some people think that they're keeping up milk supply by expressing, but it's actually the sucking action of the baby (different to that of any pump) which stimulates the best milk flow. Your physical contact gets the 'love hormone' activated. If your breastfeeding experience continues to be unsuccessful after about 12 weeks (extremely rare under normal circumstances), consider teaching your baby to take your milk from either a spoon or a cup. Again, you can tell your baby is getting enough fluids by the number of wet nappies. Be sure to keep expressing, so you can get the hindmilk with each feed.

If you *genuinely* believe you couldn't breastfeed, it will allow for inner-healing if you can do some soul-searching and seek an understanding as to why your milk didn't let down; or seek help until your navigation through difficulties, real or perceived, is revealed ~ and then share *that* as your truth when stating your breastfeeding story.

Body image Some women are worried they might lose their partner to a perkier model if they 'let themselves go' by breastfeeding. Do you really want a partner who is so shallow that he identifies you by the size and shape of your breasts, rather than the size and shape of your heart and soul?

Such a man will *not* make a good father. If he leaves you because of your breasts sagging, ol' Cupid here can tell you, without a shadow of a doubt, that he wasn't your Mr Right. At the risk of repeating myself, breast-feeding doesn't make your breasts sag ~ pregnancy does.

I'd never be driven to surgery, and would never have sacrificed having children, for the sake of a neat pair of baps on my chest! What I *have* received is a genuine respect for my body, fuelled greatly by the love and awe my children have shown to their *fountains of love*.

Can I breastfeed after breast surgery?

Although breast surgery does have an impact on the ability to produce milk, it's important to debunk the myth that breastfeeding is impossible. Unfortunately, many of the surgeons who perform these operations don't have an understanding of lactation.

The nerves in the areola play a crucial role in breastfeeding, because they trigger the hormone oxytocin. If a woman's attitude to breastfeeding is strong, passionate and determined, then with adequate support and management she'll be well equipped to breastfeed. Unless her breasts have been cut off through a mastectomy, she'll be able to make milk. As with a woman inducing lactation to breastfeed, a surgically-affected mother may not be able to produce a full breast milk supply for her baby. However, as you've read in this book, *every drop of breast milk is invaluable for a baby*.

Any woman who is willing to breastfeed, will find that many methods and aids will help her journey, regardless of her situation. The biggest issue in relation to successful breastfeeding is our psychological state. Other devices, be they chemical, mechanical or natural, are in many ways secondary to a positive attitude. Even women who aren't able to provide all of their baby's breast milk needs because of adoption or surgery, can have truly satisfying breastfeeding relationships with their children.

Always, always, *always* remember, *every* drop of milk is important.

GALACTOSEMIA ~ when Mother Nature gets it wrong, or so it seems.

When I worked as the phlebotomist (human vampire) in a hospital medical laboratory ~ another of life's jigsaw pieces ~ one of my jobs was to do heel-pricks on newborn babies. It was horrendous. I begged my boss to relieve me of this duty. It's one thing to have adults come to the lab for blood tests, but newborn babies don't ask for tests, and should never have to undergo such routine practices. The heel-prick test is to identify babies who have galactosemia. It's always a parent's choice whether to have this test. If you're in a hospital where it's routine, you can withdraw your consent. Neither of my babies had the heel-prick test.

Hospital routine was such that mothers didn't come into the nursery where the test was done. I cringe now to think of this. If a mother consents to the heel-prick test, then the very least she should do is hold her baby while it's being done. Don't abandon him while he's going through this traumatic experience.

Galactosemia is a *very* rare disease, in which a child is born without the enzyme to digest lactose. Lactose is the sugar in milk. If a baby has galacto-semia and receives lactose, he will develop irreversible brain-damage, and die. You could say, Mother Nature is covering her backside, because breast milk is the <u>only</u> food to fully develop the body and brain of a human. She knows it's not for the benefit of the human species to have a child who can't receive breast milk.

Perhaps, though, it isn't down to Mother Nature getting it wrong in the first place. Research indicates there are babies born with all sorts of conditions which *could* have been avoided if the mother <u>and</u> father had optimal dietary and lifestyle choices in the two years preceding their baby's *conception*. (See the work of Foresight for studies on pre-conception cleansing).

Enfamil® Pregestimil® is an iron-fortified, lactose-free, sucrose-free, hypoallergenic infant formula appropriate for infants with galactosemia. Although medically it's considered that galactosemia is one of those conditions where formula is actually needed, there are other options, such as making your own milk substitute.

A DIY living milk drink

All commercial formula is a static, non-living product. Some mothers, who for whatever reason, can't breastfeed, are creating their own holistic, 'living' milk. The usual combination is that of approximately half freshly-made hemp milk (rich in amino acids), freshly-made almond milk, and algae oil (pierce the capsules and pour the oil into the milk) for vital DHA. You can use fresh baby coconuts. Coconut milk was used during the Second World War as a direct substitute for blood plasma. You can sweeten the milk with home-made fresh fruit or carrot juice (don't use commercial juice as it's pasteurised and contains no enzymes).

It would be best to work with a qualified naturopath or living foods consultant in developing a breast milk replacement for your baby.

Always keep in mind what a baby needs ~ skin to skin touch, eye contact, smiles, hugs, the sound of your heartbeat and to feed from both the left and right hand side. Do everything you can to support your baby.

Adoption and breastfeeding

It's a little known fact that *any* woman can induce milk into her breasts. Women who wish to adopt a baby can choose to follow this path so he can have the best start in life. Ideally, breastfeeding would begin with a newborn, whose sucking reflex is still intact. However, with passion and commitment, there's nothing to stop a mother expressing milk for a baby, and giving it to him on a spoon or in a cup. As with breastfeeding after birth, it's important for the nipples to be stimulated. Before your baby arrives, you'll need some time to develop supply. You can begin with an electric breast pump (the dual sort is best), and pump every three hours.

A birthing woman has hormones which induce lactation. A woman who is adopting can try some different options. Commonly, a drug called domperidone is used. The drug was created for digestive problems; however, it was discovered that it makes breasts leak milk. The choice to take such a drug is a purely personal one. I wouldn't, but you have to weigh up the pros and cons yourself. If, like me, you prefer a more wholesome and natural route, you could try fenugreek seeds. It's an aniseed flavoured herb, well-known for increasing breast milk.

Some women choose to re-lactate many years after having children, either because they want to work as a wet nurse (nursing children not born to them), or to help out in areas devastated by man-made or natural disasters.

When choosing to lactate or re-lactate, pumping for twenty minutes every few hours will begin the process. You need to do this for at least a month. Have several cups of herb tea a day. You can vary your drinks between fenugreek, fennel, red raspberry leaf, comfrey and nettle.

Some adoptive mothers don't produce adequate breast milk, initially, for their baby's needs. In order to avoid nipple confusion, which arises when alternating between breast and bottle, I recommend she uses an aid that allows her to offer a supplement while baby is nursing. This is called SNS ~ Supplemental Nursing System. Essentially, it's a small bottle the mother can wear, that has a very thin tube taped to her nipple. This system works even if there is no breast milk. Clearly, though, the more the mother is able to produce breast milk, the less she'll need to provide a supplement. Depending on the age a baby is adopted, she may find it difficult to receive physical attention. Persevere. The more skin-to-skin contact you can provide, the sooner she'll settle into your family. She'll learn your voice, your touch, your family's rhythm.

A study found that the milk of women who induced lactation, compared to a birth mother's breast milk at 10 days post partum, showed little difference[60]. Any woman with undamaged breasts can induce lactation, but she will, without doubt, need determination, commitment and a great attitude. If you're planning to adopt a baby, give yourself about nine months to prepare your breasts.

The Drinks Are On Me

Reclaiming the sacred feminine

The pea-sized pituitary gland is in charge of a number of hormones, including prolactin ~ the one which stimulates breasts to make milk. Both men and women are able to lactate. It comes more easily to women when they are pregnant and breastfeeding. So, those stories you've heard about Milk Men are true! Women who believe they can't breastfeed might like to look at stimulating the pituitary gland.

Breastfeeding is truly a mind/body experience. For some women it happens with no effort, for others it takes a conscious connection with all aspects of their being before they're able to release milk fully and freely.

We can develop this part of our self; by *deliberately* choosing to become a more gentle human being ~ more kind, more forgiving. Let it become a habit. Our inner self, when developed, can lead us through the journey of life with greater awareness and consciousness, for ourselves and others. The energy the pituitary gland sends to our body can be life-affirming, or it can literally send forth 'death' hormones. Allowing ourselves to breastfeed another human being is the highest call we can ask of our body.

Oxytocin, from the Greek, meaning 'swift birth', is found naturally in the body; it is made in the hypothalamus, and lets down our milk. We can trigger the release of oxytocin through stimulation of the uterus, cervix and nipples.

Breast milk is a living food. It carries the vibrational energy of the mother who makes it, so it's vital that she goes into her parenting consciously, and aware of her role. It isn't just our mother's energy in the breast milk, but every human being in her evolutionary line. Our ancestral lineage, from the beginning of time, is contained in each baby's mother's breast milk. Breastfeeding is a holy act between mother and child. It is, in many ways, a link for the child to the Divine. Our milk gently coaxes our baby Earthside, softly beckoning her to be more fully in the human body she has chosen; and yet, it's a reminder of the Unconditional Love she experienced when she was a being of Light. Spiritually, breast milk is the nearest equivalent the human being has to Light.

Finding our heart centre

Chakras: how an ancient Hindu teaching can help with successful breastfeeding

The Indian spiritual master, Paramahansa Yogananda, wrote in his book, Man's Eternal Quest, about seven centres of life and consciousness in the spine and brain, called chakras. These spinning vortices of energy enliven not only our physical body, but our astral body, too. Having a basic understanding of these 'wheels' of life allows us to embrace a new way of being, which lets us live life fully. These wheels, or discs, radiate light and energy. They begin at the base of the spine, and can be found along its length, up to the head. They have been likened to rungs on our spiritual ladder.

From sacred, ancient teachings we learn that these discs of light allow the soul to enter and leave during meditation. Man's eternal quest is to be awakened to these centres. In many ways it's like the fast-track back Home (to the place from which we came before birth). One of the most beautiful descriptions of the chakras likens them to lotus flowers, so that when they are open, the energy of the Universe is able to travel up our spine.

These teachings have been in the west for only a short time. In Hindi, chakra means *wheel of spinning energy*. Just as each chakra responds to a colour, or light frequency, so too do they respond to musical notes. Colour therapy, and other forms of vibrational medicine, utilise the teachings of the chakras to bring alignment and energy to the body.

We are each born at different stages of spiritual development and awareness. Sometimes one or more chakras need to be awakened, and this often happens through life experiences 'opening us up', rather than people consciously waking up a chakra. Sometimes, just understanding what each chakra represents is more than enough to stimulate the energy associated with it. The process of aligning and awakening chakras is very much holistic, taking in our whole being. It happens spontaneously and naturally throughout our childhood development if our biological needs have been met. The unfolding of our physical development reaches through into our spiritual unfolding.

The red chakra, at the base of the spine, is commonly called the root chakra. This is essentially because when it's 'open', it grounds us to the Earth. We feel settled, and have no need to escape or live in fear. In its truest sense, it represents our physical survival on earth. A closed root chakra leads to a feeling of violence, mistrust, constipation and anger. It resonates to the musical note C.

Taking a step up to note D, we find the navel chakra, over the sacrum area. Orange in colour, this chakra represents our creativity. This comes in many forms, and includes our sexuality and emotions. Common imbalances include bladder problems, lower back pain, sexuality issues, health issues with the uterus, jealousy and possessiveness.

Resonating to note E is a yellow chakra which is in the solar plexus area, a little way, perhaps a couple of inches, above our navel. It's here we feel our sense of power, emotions, sensitivity. A closed or unbalanced solar plexus chakra can be seen in digestion issues, eating disorders, anger, hate, fear, and either a lack of willpower or over-use of personal power.

The green chakra, next to our heart, is where we let through peaceful feelings, love and harmonious energy into relationships. Resonating to the note F, we're very aware of this chakra when we fall in love. This is our *breastfeeding chakra*. In terms of intimate and sexual relationships, our falling in love sends energy to the chakras below, igniting feelings of sexual attraction (root chakra). When we are married, or living with a partner, this stability manifests in the solar plexus.

A closed heart chakra leads to reluctance in letting milk flow for our baby, rigidity in love, lack of compassion, anger, health issues to do with the heart, and immune-system stress. People with a well-developed heart chakra are aware of pre-conception communication with their future children. They have an ability to feel what others, including animals and plants, are feeling. The devotional love we feel for our baby, enhances and *awakens* this chakra through the constant stimulation of love. It moves us away from more worldly associations of dependent love, and onto the path of unconditional love. Our breastfeeding chakra relates to our mammalian (milk) brain. It is, indeed, the link between the human and divine and unites the lower and upper chakras. It's the basis of our spirituality and the key to our biology.

It's no exaggeration to say that in our Western world, many people's heart chakras are either closed or unbalanced. When we breastfeed our babies, our love and our milk are inseparable. Breastfeeding is on the verge of being lost to humanity, the consequences of which go way beyond damaging our collective immune system, brain development and psychological well-being. When humanity's heart centre closes down, so too will the human race. We simply can't co-exist with closed hearts indefinitely. Because this syndrome of *closed heart chakra* is so widespread, it's considered 'normal' to be distrustful and unloving. For most people, love is now expressed to only one or two people, such as a partner or children, and then it's usually only given with conditions.

Humans were designed to give and receive unconditional love from whoever they shared their lives with. At the time of writing, more than seven million people in Britain live alone, that is, more than one in eight people. This isolation and alienation is an example of closing down our heart centre. It's from here where love begins, not in our mind.

We can all learn to love again, even if we find it hard because of conditioning or our own choice to shut down the love chakra. Try practising on your cat. Borrow a pet if you don't have one. Let her lie in your lap, undisturbed, and just *feel* (don't analyse) a ray of light moving from your heart centre to hers.

Imagine a green lotus, above your heart, opening up fully, radiating with luminous light. When this flows freely, think of your favourite tree. Mine is a sycamore in our village that shows us the changing seasons with such beauty. Send love from your blossoming lotus to the tree you've chosen. Really allow yourself to feel what it's like to connect with another living being. Imagine an old friend who is dear to you. See his face up close. Smile, and again, let the light of love join your hearts together.

When we refuse to love living beings, our lives become full of addictions. These may be heartless sex, devitalised foods, compulsion to buy the latest electrical goods and clothing, watching tv, overuse of a computer, or engaging with any other item which doesn't have feelings.

Stepping up a notch to note G we find the blue chakra, in our throat area. This centre is the home of our ability to communicate and express ourselves. When we're in a place of judgement, or having difficulty saying our 'truth', then we find ourselves having health issues with the throat. The feeling of having a "lump in our throat" comes when we are holding onto our emotions there.

The beautiful colour indigo radiates from our Brow chakra, or third eye. Relating to the musical note A, it's from here we ask ourselves about the nature of reality, the spiritual purpose of our existence. When functioning well, we're intuitive, have rich and meaningful dreams, perceive Higher Truths, may have prophetic and insightful visions. Closed Brow chakras can be recognised through difficulty with eye-sight, headaches and an inability to concentrate.

The crowning glory of the chakras, sings to note B, and is violet in colour. Located at the top of the head, literally like a crown, this chakra helps us integrate our physical being with our Spiritual Self. It gives us the ability to function in this world without losing connection to our Divine Self. When we close off this chakra, it's seen in symptoms such as feeling uninspired by anything in life, and depression. Meditating or focusing on the crown chakra energises the pituitary gland. It fills you with inspiration, creativity and awareness of a higher consciousness. Breathe deeply, with eyes closed. Imagine the colour soaking over the top of your head in a crown shape. Imagine it, placed upon you.

Liquid love ~ the true meaning of breast milk

We've looked at the physical ways breast milk is made and its ingredients; however, the flow of breast milk is sourced from our *spiritual* being. When we can understand this fully, we become empowered, not only for ourselves as breastfeeding mothers, but also to help women who believe they've 'got no milk'.

Throughout history, we've associated the beginning of lactation with pregnancy and birth. However, while this may be relatively true *physically*, spiritually, anyone capable of *allowing love to flow freely* can create milk from their breasts.

The Drinks Are On Me

The milk which flows from the human breast is a physical expression of unconditional love ~ it's liquid love. Our breasts, too, are a symbol of love, sitting over the heart chakra, known in Hindi as *Anahata*. The giving of love is permanent. When a woman believes she has no milk, although we can offer mechanical, herbal and psychological support, if she's *spiritually closed* in her heart chakra (symbolic of a closed heart), then she won't *let down* the milk in her body. We mistakenly take it to mean she has 'no milk'. Such a response may be due to conditioning in a mother's own childhood, or, as some people believe, previous lives in which the person kept their heart closed. Opening our heart chakra enables our milk to flow. Deep and honest soul-searching is needed by a woman in this situation. She can heal these deep wounds.

Lactation is often induced artificially in women not going through pregnancy or birth. However, it can be triggered instantly by a deep desire to express love to a baby, or indeed any other human being. Anecdotes abound of women spontaneously lactating at the sound or sight of a baby, regardless of whether they've ever breastfed.

Our western culture places great emphasis on the physical body. Many spiritual traditions teach that we are spiritual beings having a human experience. As such, our divine heritage means we were born to love, and receive love. This is the same for every human being, regardless of religious, philosophical or spiritual outlook. So perhaps the question of creating an abundance of milk isn't "how do I make milk?", but "how do I open my heart to love?".

Do I really want to give love to my baby?

Do I know how much my baby loves me?

Am I willing to allow my baby to receive fully my love? Do I have a fear of my baby absorbing my love?

We're all at different stages of our spiritual evolution, we're all learning to love. It doesn't serve any of us to remain in victim mode. Regardless of our circumstances, we must take responsibility for our situation, and the choices and actions which have brought us to the present. When we play the role of victim, acting helpless and weak, then what started off as a temporary act, soon becomes our *permanent* state of being. This then becomes our reality.

Breast health and metaphysical interpretations

Breast cancer is rampant. Physically, there are many reasons for this. For example, tight bras are implicated in increases in breast cancer[54]. It's simply not natural to have what are essentially a couple of 'fat' glands constantly bound up in a warm environment.

When you choose your nursing bra, don't wear ones with under-wire. Try and obtain bras made from organic cotton or hemp, rather than synthetic fabrics. Your skin is a living and breathing organ. It will absorb what you hold against it. If you can, go braless as much as possible ~ you'll be doing your breasts and milk ducts a great service. Going braless leads to superior breast health. If you require breast pads, consider making your own simple ones, which can be thrown in the wash with your clothes. Avoid the plastic backed, disposable ones. Keep your nipples as dry as possible. That's the secret of a happy nipple ~ dry, dry, dry!

Breast health includes allowing sunlight on your skin, and avoiding the use of toxic chemicals from deodorants under your arms. Seek out natural alternatives. Likewise, eliminate as many toxins from your environment as possible.

However, any disharmony in the physical body is a symptom of something on an emotional level. Our body is essentially the last place it manifests. Ironically, we then try and treat the physical body rather than healing the cause.

Our breasts are symbolic of nurturing. Expressing our nurturing self in a balanced way allows us to value our self and others. Our creative life is explored with joy and happiness, and without resentment.

An imbalance can occur when we refuse to nurture, by holding back our love, either through not breastfeeding or not actively being involved in the raising of our family. We tend to feel little love or compassion for ourselves. This often is the result of not being nurtured in infancy ourselves. Another imbalance can be seen in women who 'over-nurture' and engage in 'smother-love', meaning they don't give their children, partner, friends and extended family room to breathe. This search for value and purpose within relationships creates a negative state of co-dependency.

Can you recognise yourself functioning somewhere between these extremes?

Metaphysically, which means to look beyond the physical, problems with the left breast have been associated with a refusal to nourish and nurture oneself. These are the people pleasers, always putting everyone else's needs way ahead of their own. Some people do it willingly, others with a more martyred tone, making it quite clear that it's a 'burden', but they have no choice. The irony is that these people, who are willing to do so much for others, tend to feel unloved.

At the right breast, problems manifest for those who have difficulty allowing people to live their own lives. They tend to express this through dictating relationships, being over-bearing and over-protective. Their path is to learn to trust that relationships can be safe without control; that love is given and received.

Breast problems, such as cancer, can be cut away, chased away with chemicals/radiation and other conventional treatment. Other people use complementary medicine, such as visualisation or raw food diets, for example.

The Drinks Are On Me

The true healing though, must always come from the emotional body, otherwise the issues will manifest again in a 'louder' way until the message is heard.

By following the middle path, that of balanced expression, we find our attention in the area of the heart, rather than the breasts. This is an integration of mindful awareness.

Ours is a culture which instructs women to look for lumps in their breasts each month. The unspoken message of this ritual is to *invite* the lumps in with our constant attention. What if, instead, we supported each other in acknowledging breasts as an important, beautiful, vital and expressive aspect of our being? What if, each month, we nurtured this part of our body with tender thoughts, prayer and physical care, such as massage? What if, instead of being slaves to bras for the 'ideal' of a perky breast, we enjoyed regular Pilates sessions and built up our pectoral muscles? What if we simply looked at breasts differently? Being mindful of seeing the heart area positively will help us find balance and peace.

Forgiveness

Breastfeeding is one of the most controversial subjects in the parenting field. Why is this, when it's obviously the most natural way to feed our babies? Our life is a patchwork of choices. Sometimes they lead to great outcomes and we're happy with the bed we lie in, other times, not so. For many mothers their choices appear as a mirror of suffering. On our life's path we do have times when we simply could have made other choices. It's important to honour these moments. We have to recognise, bless, and let go of the pain and trauma. It's time for all of us to reclaim the sacred feminine, to affirm our spirit self, and leave a gift for our daughters, nieces and grand daughters.

A crisis is another word for choice. In many ways it is liberating because it means we have opportunities to act and be differently. We free ourselves from debilitating psychic chains when we make the decision to let go of bitterness and resentment towards self and others. Sometimes we feel anger and resentment towards our baby for our choices, and other times those feelings are directed at those people in our lives who perhaps didn't support us adequately. We all have a story to tell. Both bottle-feeding and breastfeeding mothers may recognise themselves in these words. How often have we judged another? How often has a little part of ourselves died because we didn't follow our heart? How easy is it to tear another down to justify our own choices? We must take responsibility for ourselves, in the present moment, and provide the necessary spiritual nourishment to move forward. Both bottle-feeding mothers and breastfeeding mothers can *unite* towards a common goal ~ that of ensuring our daughters and grand-daughters are educated, nourished and supported in feeding their children naturally. We must stand up and speak.

To be in touch with the sacred feminine means we walk a path of re-birth, and awaken into a joyous and loving self. Choices which have led us down paths we'd rather not have taken must be mourned and then left behind. Honour these times as your Blessing Places. They give meaning to your journey. Let go. There's no room for ghosts, only the blossoming of climbing roses.

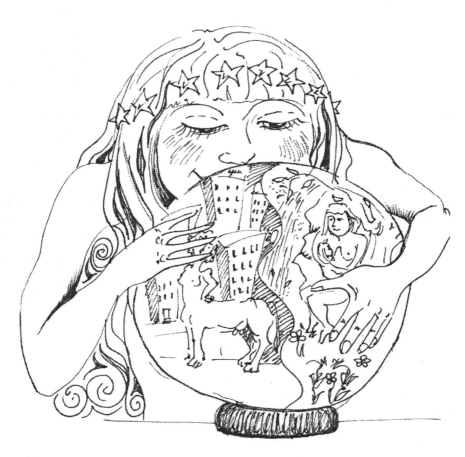

What future? Man's devolution into cow, or reclamation of breastfeeding our babies?

The Drinks Are On Me

Human milk for human babies

Many people assume infant formula is second best to breast milk. The second choice for infant feeding is a mother's own *expressed* milk. The third choice is donor breast milk. Milk donation isn't a new idea. Breast milk has been banked for about a century. A donor milk bank was first opened in 1909, in Vienna. Milk banks collect, store, screen, process and distribute breast milk donated voluntarily by a mother for feeding to premature babies or hospitalised infants with health issues.

People are often asked to carry cards showing their willingness to donate body parts after death, but it's not common knowledge that donating breast milk can save a newborn baby's life. Even a few drops of breast milk will make all the difference.

There are many cases, often in the neonatal or special care baby units, where the mother can't breastfeed her newborn or premature baby. It may be simply that her milk hasn't come in yet, or perhaps she's ill or recovering from surgery.

Donor mums need to be healthy and have a plentiful milk supply. Their milk is tested and heat treated. Just an ounce of milk will feed a premature baby for a day and a half.

Milk banks cannot accept milk from women who smoke, or use illegal drugs. All potential donors are tested for infections. Different countries have their own guidelines as to what constitutes health. Some screen more heavily, or have stricter guidelines, in relation to past blood transfusions and organ implants. It's important you aren't taking certain medications, smoking, or drinking a lot of caffeine or alcohol, have rubella or have been recently vaccinated.

Donating breast milk should occur in the early months of breastfeeding, usually before the end of six months. As little as 30 ml a day can be donated. At any given time in the UK, there are up to 200 women donating breast milk.

Milk banks exist throughout the UK and in many other countries.

A full list of all UK Milk Banks is available from:

UKAMB (United Kingdom Association of Milk Banks),
Queen Charlotte's and Chelsea Hospital,
Du Cane Rd.,
Hammersmith,
London W12 0HS

Hung out to dry

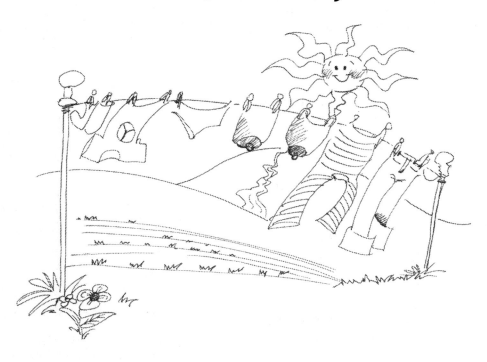

So now what? Dried up, probably empty, no longer needed ~ what's a girl to do with two retired breasts? I'm just one mum, but if I can learn about breastfeeding and share my knowledge with at least one other mum, then I'll have done my job well. We increase breastfeeding rates one baby at a time, one mum at a time.

It would be selfish to go into retirement and keep my experiences to myself. I know without a shadow of a doubt that my girls will breastfeed their own children; but is that enough after ten years of breastfeeding, given the drastic current world breastfeeding decline? Surely I can help one more woman? One more child? One more father? And if one of these people helped one other person, and that person helped another, then maybe, just maybe...

We no longer live in communities where we easily have access to other breastfeeding mothers around us. It's crazy, but that's the world we've created. Instead, we have to go to breastfeeding groups!

The Drinks Are On Me

I urge you, every time you see a woman breastfeeding, regardless of the baby's age, please *jump* out of your comfort zone and say "Congratulations for breastfeeding your baby. You're doing a great job!" It's a little random act of kindness that will have ripple (or is that nipple?) effects, for years to come. If you're too shy to say anything, make a copy of the little coupon below and leave it with her.

> ### CONGRATULATIONS
>
> *I noticed you were*
> *breastfeeding your child*
> *and I wanted to congratulate you*
> *on following your motherly intuition*
> *and doing such a great job!*

Here's my prophecy of the future: if we keep feeding the vast majority of babies on artificial milk, over the generations we will weaken, our brains won't develop as nature intended, immune systems just won't cut the mustard, and we'll die out, but probably not before we completely destroy everything around us.

We have a choice. We can take our babes in arms and breastfeed. We can pass on mammalian instincts, and fight the growing tide of cultural ignorance.

It's worth remembering the story of two leopards rescued in South Africa at two weeks of age, that were then raised on cow's milk. The poor leopards now have big heads, big tummies, and eyes open all the time. Why? They were fed the wrong milk!

What's my Utopian vision for breastfeeding around the world? For *at least* two and a half years of breastfeeding, at the breast rather than expressed milk, to be the norm; and if parent-led weaning must happen, for it to be gentle, rather than abrupt. We should make it a priority to ensure every child receives breast milk for *at least* two and a half years ~ if not from their mother, then from a relative, or a friend; for women to be more generous with their own breast milk by donating to other mums who genuinely don't have milk, are ill, or to babies who've been left without a mother.

It is only the power of love that will have us saying 'we've a great fu-ture'; that will cause us to move our feet, take action, and make great changes one step at a time. Right now, we need a spiritual revolution, a turning inward.

The positive consequences of breastfeeding cannot be overestimated. The Californian Crime Commission has failed to find one criminal who had the benefit of full-term breastfeeding or a gentle (non-medical) birth. We can't fool our biology.

Unconditional love reaches beyond the physical world and into the realm where we are capable of great feats ~ of devotion, dedication and incredi-ble creation. It reaches into our world-wide web, the threading of a hu-man's individuality into a connection of unimaginable proportions. Imagine what six billion conscious, caring, loving people could do for each other, and the home they all share? Imagine if this care and love first began at home, in the family, at the breast?

What's the future for humanity? That's your choice. Will it be of love or indifference? Whichever you choose, and it *is* a choice, it will indeed make all the difference to whether we even have a future.

Happy breastfeeding!

To find out more about holistic parenting, you might like to consider subscribing to The Mother magazine: www.themothermagazine.co.uk

or visit our publisher's website: www.artofchange.co.uk

After completing this book, I received the following article from Joseph Chilton Pearce, for inclusion in The Mother magazine. It's such an important piece of work that I feel this book would not be complete without it. I am very grateful for Joseph's permission to reprint it here in full.

Birth and Bonding
by Joseph Chilton Pearce

Shortly before scheduled to speak at a conference on birth-bonding, I received a lengthy form from The American College of Obstetricians, stating that I had to disclaim any *conflict of interest* I, as a presenter at said conference, might have with the practices of said College, my signature of agreement being required. In the ensuing paragraphs I was warned that my failure to comply would result in said College informing the audience attending my talk of such perfidy on my part. That college, consisting of some forty thousand obstetricians, had just passed a resolution that any woman desiring a c-section could have one without *any* medical reason, simply her own whims. Both hospital and obstetrician make far more money on c-section than ordinary vaginal delivery; birth accounts for some two-thirds of all hospital revenue, and a majority of hospitals are owned by large corporate chains.

Documentation for the following short essay is in the common domain, but for sake of brevity is largely left out here. I also leave out reference to the epochal work of James Prescott and Michel Odent. My intent is to cover aspects of birth-bonding not ordinarily addressed.

A Conflict between Nature's Intelligence and Human Intellect

Recall the triad of interdependent needs Paul MacLean states as imperative:
audio-visual communication
nurturing
play

All are established by mother-infant bonding at birth, and stabilised through breastfeeding in the first year of life. Deprived of bonding and breastfeeding, all subsequent development (of both infant and mother) is compromised.

Years ago, Muriel Beadle asked, "why is it that the human infant seems born in a state of alert excitement that quickly reverts to distress, followed by conscious withdrawal?" (This withdrawal lasts for ten to twelve weeks on average.) Answering Beadle's query leads to a richly woven fabric of nature's proposing and man's disposing.

First, most mammals, on preparing to give birth, seek out the most hidden, preferably dark, quiet and safe haven available. At the first sign of any intrusion - even the snapping of a twig in the wilds - the creature's natural intelligence slows, or even stops, birthing, waiting to make sure the setting is safe. We humans' mammalian instincts are in charge at birth, interpreting and responding to environmental signals. If safe, supported and secure, in touch with herself and nature, human mothers have given birth in as little as twenty minutes. But at the first sign of any interference of *any* sort, regardless of the nature or reason for it, the birthing process will be disrupted, slowed down, or even halted, by these ancient and powerful intelligences within.

If disruption does occur, a mother's smooth muscular coordination of resonant responses can be lost, and chaos reign within her - muscle fighting with muscle, instinct with instinct, inner-knowing confused by outer intrusions, nature's intentions clashing with culture's attentions, mother and infant losing on all fronts. Sadly, this has been the norm for the majority of modern women, and a primary cause of our ever increasing personal-social turmoil.

Nikos Tinbergen (Nobel laureate in ethology) studied the metabolism of the early infant, and determined that a human newborn needs to feed about every twenty minutes in its early days - the periods between, growing progressively longer as the months go by. Mother's milk, it seems, has few fats and proteins, but is, instead, as Israeli doctors termed it, a rich cocktail of hormones. This rather thin diet requires that the infant feed quite frequently - which is the whole point. Some mammals, rabbits for instance, produce a milk so heavy with fats and proteins, their offspring need only feed once or twice a day, allowing mother's forage to make more rich milk for that next powerful wallop. One might wonder why nature didn't make a similarly handy arrangement for us humans, instead of a procedure so inconvenient, particularly to us modern people. Look a bit further, however, and we find that nature did this on behalf of an intricately, interwoven fabric of interdependent needs, rather exclusively human and absolutely critical to being *fully* human.

First, hydrochloric acid - found abundantly in other infant mammals, since necessary for the digestion of fats and proteins, is not found in human infants in the same quantity, since so few fats and proteins are found in human mothers' milk *[author's note: not to be confused with essential fatty acids]*. Some nine months after birth, however, hydrochloric acid spontaneously appears in full flow. Remember this nine-month marker in what follows here: just as it took nature nine months to grow that infant in mother's womb in the first place, it takes another nine months in the <u>arms</u> of that mother to firmly establish the infant in the matrix of its new world, continue the growth of the infant's brain, and stabilise its body functions, particularly the heart; and nature does what she can to keep that infant 'in-arms' for that period.

The Drinks Are On Me

Audio-visual is number one in MacLean's Triad of Needs, and a rudimentary hearing develops early in utero.

If the foetus has normal hearing and a speaking mother, language development gets underway in the second trimester, through muscular responses the infant makes to phonemes, those foundational units of words in the mother's speech. This language foundation builds in successive stages until birth, and leads to speech.

Vision, however, while it occupies more of our brain than all other senses put together, obviously can't develop in utero (though visual sensitivity appears early on, as seen in an infant's aversion to bright lights should we shine them directly on the mother's belly - which prompts the infant to turn its head away). Visual *development*, though, and the audio-visual communication that accompanies it, must await birth to unfold. (There is a vast difference between stimuli and communication.)

And at birth, if given a *face* within six to twelve inches away, two immediate responses take place in the newborn: its initial excited alertness (noted by Muriel Beadle long ago) stabilises, and visual, and audio-visual, development begin. That close-up face literally turns on the infant brain, its conscious awareness, and keeps it turned on. For the infant is born with a pre-set neural pattern for cognising-perceiving a face, and will lock eyes on a face if one is given at that required distance, and hold that face in focus. Perception-cognition automatically begins, activating the infant's entire body-brain system. Focus is immediate, so long as a face is there to focus on; parallax (muscle coordination of the eyes) forms within minutes (so the infant can even follow that face around should it move about), and a construction of knowledge (of a visual world begins) - a world based on this stable foundation of a face. Before long, other objects in the mother's immediate vicinity are registered, and, through processes of association, corresponding new neural patterns form, and a cognitive field of recognisable objects grows exponentially (as does the brain itself) - so long as that face-pattern remains the <u>stable point</u> of reference. Although any face will work at birth, face *constancy* and all that goes with it, is the critical factor in this early infant movement from known to unknown, and vitally necessary for a stable and stress-free development.

Should a face *not* be presented, along with all the attendant functions accompanying it (to be described shortly), distress takes over and conscious awareness will fade within about 45 minutes, and does not ordinarily reappear, as mentioned above, for upwards of some ten to twelve weeks on average.

Bonding as a reciprocal function between mother and infant is then fragmented, and the ongoing nurturing instincts which bonding awakens and locks into the mother's responses aren't there. Most infants then receive only sporadic exposures to a face or faces, and by then, consciousness largely retreated, the awareness needed for such cognition to take place and be stabilised is missing. Nature will compensate as best she can, but under these conditions, her capacity to compensate is diminished and slow.

Nature arranged that this magical face-trigger be some six to twelve inches from those equally wonderful mammary glands, from which flows that life-giving fat-and-protein-free nurturing-nourishment. Nursing on cue assures a frequent reinforcing of the stable face pattern on which vision and awareness are based. 'Object constancy', as Piaget called it, the stabilisation of an object-world of vision, occurs around the ninth month of this busy construction period. Among the many facets of this ninth-month milestone, myelination of the neural patterns of this primary visual world takes place, making the neural foundations permanent, and cheap to operate, the ongoing expansion of the visual world automatic and effortless. Now nature can turn her world-building energy to other developments, which open around that pivotal ninth month. (Any society separating mothers from infants at birth will have a disproportionately large population with impaired vision. The United States, for instance, is virtually a nation of eyeglasses. (We ignore and/or forget pre-literate, primitive people have far more accurate and extensive vision than we have - some of those people can see the rings of Saturn with their naked eye). Far more seriously, for those willing to look, note how many of the infant-toddlers we see, pushed about in various wheeled devices that keep them separate, out of the way and helpless, have strangely vacant, barely-focused eyes, and vapid, nobody-at-home expressions - as though a light were blown out in their brain, or rather, *never ignited.*

Some forty years ago, Whittlestone, at The University of Adelaide, pointed out that the mother's heart is a most critical factor from conception through birth. This has been well established. Now we know that her heart is every bit as critical a part of the next nine-months in-arms. Over half a century ago, researchers found that a heart cell could be removed from a live rodent's heart, put in an appropriate nutrient to keep it alive, and, when examined through a microscope, would continue to pulsate, expanding and contracting regularly, according to the rhythm set by the donor-heart. After some time of this separation from the heart, however, that rhythmic pulsation would deteriorate until collapse, and that erratic jerky spasm called fibrillation, precursor to death of the cell, would set in. If two heart cells are placed on the slide, however, separated from each other, when fibrillation begins, through bringing the two cells into close proximity with each other (they do not have to touch and can be separated by a tiny barrier) they both stopped their death-spasms and re-established their co-ordinated pulsation, in sync with each other. Each cell had 'lifted the other' out of that fibrillation that leads to death, into the shared rhythm of life. This miracle occurs, it turns out, through bringing into spatial conjunction the electro-magnetic fields that arise from, and surround, each heart cell, a phenomenon only recently discovered. These electro-magnetic (EM) fields are not affected by ordinary physical boundaries, and when the fields come into contact, their waves entrain, go into the same coherent pattern (and coherent wave-forms reinforce each other).

This coherent resonance, in turn, lifts those cells out of chaos into order. Cells and their EM fields mutually give rise to and/or influence each other, and the same phenomenon occurs, on a far larger and far more serious level, with infant-mother hearts at birth, a major but largely unrecognised factor in bonding. The heart itself produces a very powerful EM field, in three successive waves: the first, and most powerful, surrounds the person's body, flooding every cell and neuron of that body; the second extends out some three feet in all directions and interacts with other heart fields within that proximity, a principal ingredient of emotion and interpersonal relationships; the third extends out indefinitely, for all purposes universally (possibly a factor or aspect of the human spirit). So at birth, following separation, infant and mother's hearts must be brought into immediate proximity, wherein they confirm and stabilise each other or 'lift' each other into their familiar, stabilised order. Again, that six-to-twelve inch distance of the mother's face, giving immediate proximity to those nurturing breasts, which are vital to the ongoing awakening experience of the newborn, assures a return to, and ongoing stabilisation of, the infant's heart, given by the mother's heart ~ the resonance of which, the infant had imprinted on it at a cellular level from conception. This order must be **continually** reinforced through that warm proximity for about a nine month period. By that time the infant heart has matured enough to 'stand on its own' without so frequent a stabilisation by mother's heart. Thus here we have another critical ninth-month milestone marker.

Newborns and mothers wired up for heart and brain wave recordings (electrocardiograms and electroencephalograms) show coherency and entrainment (matching of the wave frequencies) when infant and mother are together. Both systems become incoherent (chaotic) if prolonged separation takes place, whereupon cortisol is released by both mother and child systems, and general stress takes place. Remember our two heart cells on that microscope's slide, and *remember that excess cortisol is quite toxic to neural systems*, particularly new ones. (Remember, also, that any society interfering with natural bonding at birth will have a corresponding increase of heart trouble. When primary heart connections fail to take place, heart development in the infant is immediately compromised, and a 'wounded heart' trauma takes place in the mother, *whether she is aware of it or not*. The post-partum blues that often follows birth-separation can be a devastating experience, affecting the health of both parties thereafter.)

Years ago, biologist-anthropologist Ashley Montague wrote a now-classic work called <u>Touching</u>, and recently Mariana Caplan wrote a similar work called <u>Untouched.</u> Both are well-documented studies showing the critical necessity of infant skin-stimulus at birth. For at birth, the newborn's nervous system is quite undeveloped, since the millions of sensory nerve endings distributed over the body can't be activated or developed in utero.

In that water world, the infant's body is protected by a water-proof coating of a fatty substance called vernix caseous, the protection of which also insulates the myriad nerve endings. So at birth, all mammalian mothers vigorously lick their infants off and on for many hours, even sporadically for days thereafter, to *activate* the dormant sensory nerve endings and the peripheral nervous system, which is, of course, a primary extension of the brain.

Failure to activate these nerve endings results in a de-sensitisation affecting the reticular activating system of the old brain, where all sensory stimuli are collated or organised into those resonant patterns which are then sent on to higher cortical areas of the brain for world-making and experiencing. Touch deprivation results in a compromised and diminished over-all neural growth, sensory system and general conscious awareness in the infant, as well as affecting inner ear development, balance, spatial patterning and so on, later. (Mothers separated from their infants at birth obviously can't provide this touch-stimulus, nor are they stimulated to do so later if the separation is prolonged. Mother, too, has a critical window of opportunity for activating those ancient nurturing responses, considered by Paul MacLean to be our species survival instincts. These instincts are activated by her skin to skin contact with her infant, making bonding a reciprocal dynamic of awaking and discovery.)

Language learning, as mentioned, begins late in the second trimester as muscular responses the infant makes to the phonetic content of the mother's speech. This dynamic continues after birth, *if* the appropriate model-stimulus is provided - a speaking mother in close proximity. And, recall, during that initial nine-months of continued language learning and phonetic completion, speech preparation takes place. Around the ninth month after birth, the average infant's speech preparations have led into lalling or infant-babbling, and even the first words - if, and only if, of course, the appropriate model-signal-stimuli are provided in that critical second-matrix period, a provision made by simply nursing the infant and speaking. (Infants separated from their mothers and confined to various forms of ongoing separation thereafter [as most modern infants are - through cribs, bassinets, carriages, playpens, strollers, etc., or that most immediate and thorough devastation called day-care], are denied all these responses, and their development is correspondingly compromised. Nature will compensate as best she can - but compensation is always a poor substitute for natural, spontaneous mimetic growth.

We live in a compensated society, however, where the abnormal has been sustained until it has become the norm - we citizen-victims, none the wiser.)

Finally (in this brief survey), and perhaps the most important of all these ninth-month-markers, we come to the pre-frontal cortex, a major neural system which cannot unfold in utero (except in a most rudimentary form), and must await birth to begin its full cellular growth. If conditions are right, it will develop into the largest neural lobe.

The Drinks Are On Me

During the in-arms and early crawling period, the primary phase of pre-frontal growth takes place, completing in that significant ninth month. (A second growth spurt, equally 'experience dependent', is designed to begin at mid-adolescence. This later prefrontal growth-spurt is critically dependent on the successful completion of the first one, years before.) Since the mid 1980s, the pre-frontal cortex has been the subject of intense investigation, and is now recognised as the latest evolutionary neural system to develop (it is probably less than 50,000 years old, compared to millions up to hundreds of millions of years behind the older lobes and modules of our brain).

This latest and greatest of nature's neural achievements proves to be the executive brain, able to moderate and control all responses, reactions and instincts of those older animal brains, with their sensory-motor, defensive, sexual and instinct-bound patterns, as well as the neo-cortex giving us speech and a vastly higher intellect.

Only this newest pre-frontal system can organise the entire brain into a smoothly synchronous attention or intention, link all our lower instincts, as well as thinking-feeling, with higher fields of intelligence, and translate all the higher human attributes such as love, empathy, care, and creativity, into daily action. The pre-frontal cortex gives us what Elkhonon Goldberg rightly calls 'civilised mind' ~ if developed.

But, as Allen Schore's research makes clear, the genetic structure of the pre-frontal cortex proves to be the most 'experience-dependent' of all brain systems - that is, those genetic systems are critically dependent on appropriate environmental feedback. This feedback is given through the multi-leveled functions of infant-mother bonding and ongoing relations, and the overall positive emotional environment that should result. This feedback includes nurturing through breastfeeding, sufficient movement and sensory stimuli, immediate proximity to the mother's face and heart, the continual coherent resonance between mother and infant heart fields, language and speech stimuli, and so on.

Failure to provide this overall emotional support inevitably means a compromised pre-frontal cortex. It literally cannot grow sufficient cellular structures and make the necessary neural connections with the rest of the brain for full operation. And a compromised pre-frontal cortex results in an impaired 'emotional intelligence', with a corresponding difficulty in relating with others or controlling our ancient sexual-survival reflexes, with a corresponding tendency toward apathy, hopelessness, despair, and/or any of the many forms of violence. Just as it took nature nine months to grow the basic 'triune brain' unfolding in utero, this pre-frontal growth takes the nine months following birth, with all the attendant developments which centre around the heart. Thus all these strands, briefly sketched in the above, gather to completion around this ninth month milestone.

Then, if the necessary foundations are in place and functional, from the ninth to twelfth month another major neural structure grows to connect this new evolutionary executive brain with the ancient limbic or emotional brain, which older system has direct unmediated neural connections with the heart (through the ancient amygdale, which is as much the top part of the defensive hind-brain as lowest part of the emotional brain). Thus this orbito-frontal loop, as it is called, a large bridge between old and new, proves, as the research of Allen Schore clearly shows, the most decisive factor of our life, and is, again, critically experience dependent.

If emotional nurturing is lacking, this bridge will be compromised and/or largely de-constructed in the little development made. At this ninth-month point, when the orbito-frontal loop begins its massive growth, the ancient cerebellum, in the back of the brain, undergoes a corresponding growth spurt. The cerebellum, rudimentary until this time, since only sparsely employed, is involved in all speech, walking, coordination of muscular systems and much more. (This muscle coordination takes place through the muscle spindle system, tiny neural extensions found on each striation of muscle tissue throughout the body. These spindles played a major role in the uterine infant's physical response to those phonemes underlying language, literally 'embedding' language in the body.)

So, at this ninth-month period, as nature prepares to organise the entire forebrain into a single coherent whole, the cerebellum readies the infant body for that upright stance we humans enjoy, which will be followed by walking and talking, displayed in that excited exploration of 'building structures of knowledge' of our physical world. Infancy comes to an end, and the early child or toddler appears.

To prepare for the toddler's excited charging out to explore all aspects of the world, (equally dictated and orchestrated by nature's agenda), the child will not only touch, but taste, every item of interest in that world; and to prepare for the new diet-world opening, which will no doubt contain fats and proteins, the appropriate digestive juices are forthwith provided. Nature dutifully turns on that long-absent hydrochloric acid in the child's metabolic system. Hydrochoric acid simply wasn't needed - at least not according to millennia of genetic encoding - in that critical 'in-arms' period, for which nature provides a vastly superior food and supreme method of dispensing.

So we have now come full circle in this brief sketch of birth and bonding, its ways and means and whys, from the initial enigma of no hydrochloric acid to its grand entrance as cued by nature, when the curtain rises on a new stage of development, ushering in an ongoing series of new bondings with new matrices over the years ~ the family, the earth itself, society, the pair bonding leading to species renewal, bonding with one's own offspring, with the spirit within and universal without, and so on.

Marshal Klaus spoke of an interlocking cascade of redundant patterns nature has built in to assure this critical first bonding between mother and infant, which meets the threefold need MacLean referred to, truly an 'eternal golden braid' (to steal Hostadter's phrase). Marshal Klaus calls bonding the establishment of the greatest love affair in the universe, on which this wondrous unfolding of human life depends. Now we can see the astonishing and thorough intelligence and careful planning, the intricate interweaving of myriad critically timed and interdependent responses which nature evolved over eons of time, and invested in this birth-bonding process entrusted to us. And now, more than ever, we can see the astonishing extent to which modern practices have by-passed, compromised, or outright eliminated, virtually every item on the agenda of this incredible architectural design. Now we can understand why our medical interferences with birth - taken as axiomatic and unconsciously accepted as the norm by virtually the entire globe - are proving to be our global undoing. You cannot do to a living organism what we are now doing to the vast majority of human infants (and the ongoing spillover into the general abandonment and neglect of children taking place world-wide), without paying a price.

The ruinously expensive take-over of all birthing by hospital-medical procedures, has brought into play an equally huge and expensive cradle-to-grave therapeutic operation, undertaken in our efforts to repair the damage we are blindly causing at the same time. We witness the strange contradiction of being madly caught up in patchworks of healing and hoped-for wholeness, while blindly allowing a radically damaging, unnatural birth practice to continue unquestioned and unchecked. Our contradiction overwhelms us, neutralises our very effort at recovery, and breakdown is widespread. Child abuse and child suicide are but the most blatant signs of the breeding ground for violence our interventions are spreading worldwide.

There may never have been a 'golden age' of birthing and child rearing (the closest being the Yequanna Jean Leidloff wrote about), but also there are no historical precedents for a species abandoning its own offspring, as witnessed today, worldwide. There is a direct correlation between the final abolition of breastfeeding through an insane birthing, and *daycare* culture. Daycare, now so massively present, is but cosmetically camouflaged abandonment, and a direct result of failure of bonding. A bonded mother does not abandon her infant, no matter how socially sanctioned such behaviour might be.

Hospital-medical childbirth, now made sacrosanct, and unquestioned on every hand, is a more insidious and devious danger than atomic bombs or germ warfare, since it is unrecognised and even *unrecognisable* for the demonic force it is by the public at large. Taking away a woman's rights over her own reproductive process has been a disaster, but intervening in, and all but abolishing, the bonding of mother with infant at birth is a devastating crime against nature; perhaps the most criminal and destructive act on the planet today, and an ultimate, if slow but sure, instrument for species' suicide.

Until we get medical-hospital interference completely out of birthing, and put birth back into the hands of women and the mother herself, as nature intended, we will continue to decline as a species. Surely, the 'collective cultural imperative' for medical intervention is enormous and powerful. And surely, our entire culture promotes the medical myth through film, literature, the daily news, schooling, on and on.

But, no organisation has as yet really set about exposing the medical myth of birth, and at least trying to awaken the general public to the outrage. The focus must be put on prevention of the travesty, not therapeutic patch-work after the fact.

Surely, the medical-myth is woven into every fibre of the social fabric, but that fabric is becoming our shroud. We can awaken in future mothers the ancient intelligence of the heart; de-condition her culturally imprinted self-doubt and fear; and restore in her the knowledge and power of *being* the mother of our race, with the courage to act accordingly. In undertaking such a restoration, we will unfold an ongoing educational agenda not only for survival, but for a higher, nobler, more compassionate way of life.

Reprinted from The Mother magazine, Sept/Oct 2007, issue twenty four.

About Joseph:

Joseph Chilton Pearce has been probing the mysteries of the human mind for nearly half a century. One of his overriding passions remains the study of what he calls the "unfolding" of intelligence in children.

He is a self-avowed iconoclast, unafraid to speak out against the myriad ways in which contemporary western culture fails to nurture the intellectual, emotional, and spiritual needs and yearnings of our young people. Part scholar, part scientist, part mystic, part itinerant teacher, Pearce keeps in close touch with the most brilliant men and women in each field. He creates a unique synthesis of their work and translates the results into a common language.

World-renowned thinker, author, and advocate of evolutionary child-rearing practices, Pearce has expertise that spans a broad range of disciplines: psychology, anthropology, biology, and physics.

He is a seminal figure in the study of human consciousness and child development. His bestseller, *Magical Child*, is an exhaustive and visionary approach to child rearing, focused on support for non-violent birthing. Joseph has written and lectured internationally on human development, and the changing needs of children.

Joseph's books include:

Magical Child
Plume Books

From Magical Child to Magical Teen
Park Street Press

Magical Parent, Magical Child:
The Art of Joyful Parenting
North Atlantic Books

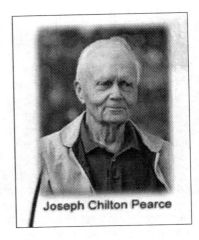
Joseph Chilton Pearce

The Biology of Transcendence:
A Blueprint of the Human Spirit
Park Street Press

The Crack in the Cosmic Egg:
New Constructs of Mind and Reality
Park Street Press

Evolution's End:
Claiming the Potential of Our Intelligence
HarperSanFrancisco

Milk banks

Countries with Milk Banks
Brazil, Bulgaria, Czech Republic, Denmark, Finland, France, Germany, Greece, India, Japan, Norway, Sweden, Switzerland, UK, Australia, Northern America.

Special Care Baby Unit,
Huddersfield Donor Breast milk Bank,
Huddersfield Royal Infirmary,
Acre Street,
Lindley, Huddersfield HD3 3EA
Contact name: Paula Wood
Fax: 01484 347249

The Human Milk Bank,
Unit 2,
The Cornsheads,
Mill Street,
Irvinestown,
Co. Fermanagh BT94 1GR
Contact name: Anne McCrea
Phone: 028 686 28333 (UK)
048 686 28333 (EIRE)

The Milk Bank,
Queen Charlotte's and Chelsea Hospital,
Du Cane Rd.,
London W12 0HS
Contact Name: Gillian Weaver, Milk Bank Manager
Phone: 020 8383 3559

Countess of Chester Hospital,
Liverpool Road,
Chester,
Cheshire CH2 1UL
Contact Name: Lynda Coulter
Phone: 01244 366416
Fax: 01244 365702

The Wirral Mothers' Milk Bank,
Clatterbridge Hospital,
Bebington,
Wirral CH63 4JY
Contact Name: Annie Atkinson
Phone: 0151 334 4000 Ext 5000
Fax: 0151 604 7138

Guy's and St Thomas' NHS Foundation Trust,
Lambeth Palace Road, London
SE1 7EH
Contact Name: Camilla Kingdon
Phone: 02071884030/1

Princess Royal University Hospital,
Infant Feeding Resource Centre,
Orpington,
Kent BR6 8ND
Contact Name: Karen Lewis & Jean Rae
Phone: 01689 864924

NICU
Medway Maritime Hospital,
Windmill Road,
Gillingham,
Kent ME7 5NY
Contact Name: Maureen Mallard
Phone: 01634 825125

Birmingham Women's Hospital Milk Bank,
Birmingham Women's Health Care NHS Trust,
Metchley Park Road,
Edgbaston,
Birmingham B15 2TG
Contact Name: Heather Barrow or Jenny Harris
Phone: 0121 472 1377 ext 4040

King's College Hospital,
The Newborn Unit, (Frederic Still Ward),
4th Floor, Golden Jubilee Wing,
King's College Hospital,
Denmark Hill,
Camberwell,
London SE5 9RS
Contact Name: Paula Blanchette
Phone: 020 7346 3038

The Drinks Are On Me

Neonatal Unit
Addenbrooke's NHS Trust,
The Rosie Hospital,
Robinson Way,
Cambridge CB2 2SW
Contact Name: Natalie Rea
Phone: 01223 245853

Oxford Human Milk Bank,
John Radcliffe Hospital,
Oxford OX3 9DU
Contact Name: Sally Inch
Phone: 01865 221695

Southampton Human Milk Bank,
Princess Anne Hospital,
Coxford Rd.,
Southampton,
Hants. SO16 5YA
Contact Name: Anita Holloway
Phone: 023 8079 6009

St Peter's Hospital Milk Bank,
Ashford & St Peter's Hospitals NHS Trust
NICU, St Peter's Hospital,
Guildford Road,
Chertsey,
Surrey KT16 0PZ
Contact Name: Suzanne Timms/Angela
Weller
Phone: 01932 722667

St George's Hospital,
Neonatal Unit,
Blackshaw Road,
Tooting,
London SW17 0QT
Contact Name: Theresa Alexander
Phone: 020 8725 1936

The Queen Mother's Hospital,
The Milk Bank, Paediatric Dept.,
The Queen Mother's Hospital,
York Hill, Glasgow G3 8SJ
Contact Name: Rhona Robinson
Phone: 0141 201 0528

Kingston Hospital,
Galsworthy Road,
Kinston Upon Thames,
Surrey KT2 7QB
Contact Name: Anna Collett
Phone: 020 8974 5390

AUSTRALIA
Mothers Milk Bank,
level 1 Office 1D,
John Flynn Private Medical Centre.
Mailing Address:
PO Box 806,
Banora Point,
NSW Australia 2486

Marea Ryan - Director -
marea@mothersmilkbank.com.au
Jenny Jones - Director, Early Childhood
Midwife and Lactaton Consultant (IBCLC)
jenny@mothersmilkbank.com.au
Kacey Patrick - Marketing Director -
kacey@mothersmilkbank.com.au
Lisa Nielsen - Secretay and ABA repre-
sentive
lisa@mothersmilkbank.com.au

- 0439 749408
Marea Mobile: 0413727545

MICHIGAN
Bronson Mothers' Milk Bank,
601 John St. Box 306
Kalamazoo, MI 49007
Phone (269) 341-8849
FAX (269) 341-8918

NEW ENGLAND
Mothers' Milk Bank of New England,
(developing)
PO Box 600091,
Newtonville, MA 02460

CALIFORNIA
Mothers' Milk Bank,
751 South Bascom Ave.,
San Jose, CA 95128
www.milkbansj.org

COLORADO
Mothers' Milk Bank at
Presbyterian St. Luke's Medical Center,
1719 E. 19th Ave.,
Denver, CO 80218
www.bestfedbabies.org

DELAWARE
Mothers' Milk Bank,
Christiana Hospital,
4755 Ogletown-Stanton Road,
Newark, DE 19718
Phone (302)733-3320

INDIANA
Indiana Mothers' Milk Bank, Inc.,
Methodist Medical Plaza II,
6820 Parkdale Place, Suite 109,
Indianapolis, IN 46254
Phone (317) 329-7146
www.immilkbank.org

IOWA
Mother's Milk Bank of Iowa,
Department of Food and Nutrition Services,
University of Iowa Hospitals and Clinics,
Room C330 GH,
200 Hawkins Drive,
Iowa City, IA 52242

NORTH CAROLINA
WakeMed Mothers' Milk Bank and Lactation Center,
3000 New Bern Ave.,
Raleigh, NC 27610

Phone (919) 350-8599

OHIO
Mothers' Milk Bank of Ohio,
Grant Medical Center @
Victorian Village Health Center,
1087 Dennison Avenue,
Columbus, OH 43201
Phone (614) 544-0811

TEXAS
Mothers' Milk Bank at Austin,
900 E. 30th St., Suite 214,
Austin, TX 78705
Phone (512) 494-0800
www.mmbaustin.org

Mothers' Milk Bank of North Texas,
1300 W. Lancaster Suite 108,
Ft. Worth, TX 76102
Phone (817) 810-0071
Toll-free 1 (866) 810-0071
www.mmbnt.org

CANADA
BRITISH COLUMBIA
BC Women's Milk Bank,
C & W Lactation Services,
4500 Oak Street, IU 30,
Vancouver, BC V6H 3N1
Phone (604) 875-2282

The Drinks Are On Me

Recommended reading

Magical child
by Joseph Chilton Pearce

The Continuum Concept
by Jean Liedloff

The politics of breastfeeding
by Gabrielle Palmer

Birth and breastfeeding
by Michel Odent

Breastfeeding matters
by Maureen Minchin

Breast milk: a natural immunisation
by Joanna Karpasea-Jones

Breastfeeding: bio-cultural perspectives
by Katherine Dettwyller and P.S MacAdam

Defining your own success: breastfeeding after breast reduction surgery
by Diana West.

The breastfeeding answer book
by Nancy Mohrbacher

Children's books about breastfeeding

Saturday with Mez: a day in the life of a breastfeeding toddler
by Lauren Serafin, Jason Rohrer, and Mez.
A unique, gorgeous board book full of wonderful black and white photos of
a toddler's breastfeeding day. Beautiful!

Near Mama's Heart
by Colleen Newman
ISBN 141207919—5
This is a full colour book with photographs of various mothers breastfeeding. The text reminds us of why breastfeeding is so wonderful.

My breastfeeding memories

The Drinks Are On Me

My breastfeeding notes

My breastfeeding notes

The Drinks Are On Me

My breastfeeding notes

My breastfeeding notes

The Drinks Are On Me

Footnotes

[1]
Anderson, G. C. (1977). The mother and her newborn: Mutual caregivers. Journal of Obstetric, Gynecologic, and Neonatal Nursing,6(5), 50-57.

Anderson, G.C. (1989). Risk in mother-infant separation postbirth. Journal of Nursing Scholarship, 21, 196-199.

Anderson G. C. (1991). Current Knowledge About Skin to Skin (Kangaroo) care for Preterm Infants. *Journal of Perinatology*, X1, (3), 216-226.

Charpak N., Ruiz-Pelaez J.G., Figueroa de C Z., & Charpak Y. (2001). A Randomised Controlled Trial of Kangaroo Mother Care: Results of Follow Up at 1 Year of Corrected Age, *Pediatrics*, 108, (5), 1072-1079.

Dragovich, D., Tamburlini, G., Alisjahbana, A., Kambarami, R., Karagulova, J., Lincetto, O., et al. (1997). Thermal control of the newborn: knowledge and practice of health professionals in seven countries. Acta Paediatrica,, 86, 645-650.

Feldman R., Eidelman A.I., Sirota L., & Weller A. (2002). Comparison of Skin to Skin (Kangaroo) and Traditional Care: Parenting Outcomes and Preterm Development. *Pediatrics*, 110, (1).

Harrison H. (1993). The Principles for Family-Centred Neonatal Care. *Pediatrics*. 92, (5), 643-650.

Keefe, M. (1987). Comparison of neonatal sleep-wake patterns in nursery versus rooming-in environments. Nursing Research, 36 (3), 140-144.

Kennell J.H. (1999). The Humane Neonatal Care Initiative. *Acta Paediatrica* 88, (4), 367-370.

Levin A. (1994). The Mother-Infant Unit at Tallinn Children's Hospital, Estonia: A Truly Baby-Friendly Unit. *Birth* (21) March.

Ludington-Hoe, S.M. and Golant, S.K. (1993). *Kangaroo Care: The Best You Can Do for Your Premature Infant*. New York: Bantam Books.

Ludington-Hoe S.M., Anderson G.A., & Hollingsead A. (1999). Birth-Related Fatigue in 34-36 Week Preterm Neonates: Rapid Recovery With Very Early Kangaroo (skin to skin) Care. *Journal of Obstetric, Gynecologic, and Neonatal Nursing*, 28, (1), 94-103.

Meier, P., & Anderson, G.C. (1987). Responses of small preterm infants to bottle and breast-feeding. American Journal of Maternal Child Nursing, 12, 97-104.

Odent Michel, Primal Health, Understanding the critical period between conception and the first birthday. Clairview Books 2002

Peters, K.C. (1992). Does routine nursing care complicate the physiologic state of the premature infant with respiratory distress syndrome? Journal of Perinatal and Neonatal Nursing, 6, 67-84.

Wilkerson, N., & Barrows, T. (1988). Synchronizing care with mother baby rhythms. American Journal of Maternal Child Nursing, 13, 264-269.

www.kangaroomothercare.com

2

Ackerman B & Tillinghast K. The Physiologic and Neurobehavioral Effects of a Single Cup Feeding on 10 Healthy Preterm Infants: Pilot Study Results. Personal Jan 1999

Howard C. Physiologic Stability of Infants During Cup and Bottle Feeding. Academy of Breastfeeding Medicine Meeting, Nov 7, 1998, Kansas City, MS

Marinelli K. Safety of Cup vs. Bottle Feedings in Premature Breastfed Infants. Academy of Breastfeeding Medicine Meeting, Nov 7, 1998, Kansas City, MS

Meier P & Anderson GC. Responses of small preterm infants to bottle and breast-feeding. MCN: American Journal of Maternal Child Nursing 1987; 12(2): 97-105

Plancoulaine-S et al. "Infant-feeding patterns are related to blood cholesterol concentration in prepubertal children aged 5-11y." *European Journal of Clinical Nutrition.* Feb 2000; 54 (2) : 114-119.

Phillips RM, Chantry CJ, Gallagher MP. Analgesic effects of breast-feeding or pacifier use with maternal holding in term infants. *Ambul Pediatr.* 2005 Nov-Dec;5(6):359-64

Marino BL et al. "Oxygen saturations during breast and bottle feedings in infants with congenital heart disease." *J Pediatr Nurs* 1995 Dec;10(6):360-4

Tully SB et al. "Abnormal tympanography after supine bottle feeding." *J Pediatr* 1995 Jun;126 (6):S105-11 Supine bottle feeding has a significant effect on middle-ear pressure dynamics, probably caused by the aspiration of milk into the ear.

3

American Academy of Pediatrics Work Group on Breastfeeding. Breastfeeding and the use of human milk. *Pediatrics* 1997;100:1035-39.

Anderson, J.W. et al. Breast-feeding and cognitive development: A meta-analysis. *Am J Clin Nutr* 1999;70:525-35

Birch E et al. Breast-feeding and optimal visual development, Journal of Ophthalmology and Strabismus, 30: 33-38, 1993.

Daniels, M. C., and L. S. Adair. Breastfeeding influences cognitive development in Filipino children. *J Nutr* 2005; 135:2589-95.

Duncan B et al. Exclusive breast-feeding for at least 4 months protects against otitis media, Pediatrics, 91(5): 867-872, 1993.

Fergusson, D, M. et al. Breast-feeding and cognitive development in the first seven years of life. *Sci Med* 1982; 16:1705-08.

Fergusson, D.M. et al. Breastfeeding and subsequent social adjustment in six- to eight-year-old children. *J Child Psychol Psychiat* 1987;28(3):378-86.

Horwood LJ et al. Breast milk feeding and cognitive ability at 7-8 years. *Arch Dis Child Fetal Neonatal Ed* 2001;84:F23-F27

The Drinks Are On Me

Horwood, L.J., Breastfeeding and later cognitive and academic outcomes. *Pediatrics* 1998;101 (1)e9

Johnson DL et al. Breastfeeding and children's intelligence. *Psych Reports* 1996;79:1179-85

Labbok MH and Hendershot GE. Does breastfeeding protect against malocclusion? An analysis of the 1981 child health supplement o the National Health Interview Survey, American Journal of Preventive Medicine, 3(4): 227-232, 1987.

Lanting, D.I., Fidler, V. Huisman, M., Touwen, B.C., Boersma, E.R. (1994). Neurological differences between 9-year old children fed breast-milk or formula-milk as babies. (1994). *Lancet*. Nov 12 344(8933):1319-22.

Lucas A et al. Breast milk and subsequent intelligence quotient in children born preterm, The Lancet, 339: 261-264, 1993.

Lucas, A. et al. A randomised multicentre study of human milk versus formula and later development in preterm infants. *Arch Dis Child* 1994;70:F141-F146

Lucas, A. et al. Randomized trial of early diet in preterm babies and later intelligence quotient. *BMJ* 1998;317(171):1481-87

Morley R. et al. Mother's choice to provide breast milk and developmental outcome. *Arch Dis Child* 1988

Mortensen EL et al. The association between duration of breastfeeding and adult intelligence. *JAMA* 02-5-8;287(18):2365-71

Morrow-Tlucak, M. et al. Breastfeeding and cognitive development in the first 2 years of life. *Soc Sci Med* 1988

Pisacane A et al. Breast-feeding and urinary tract infection, Journal of Pediatrics, 120(1): 87-89, 1992.

Pollock, J.I. Long-term associations with infant feeding in a clinically advantaged population of babies. *Dev Med Child Neurol* 1994;36(5):429-40

Reynolds A. The evidence for breastfeeding: Breastfeeding and brain development. *Ped Clin NA* 01-2;48(1):159-71

Rogan WJ and Gladen BC. Breast-feeding and cognitive development, Early Human Development, 31: 181-193, 1993.

Temboury MC et al. Influence of breast-feeding on the infant's intellectual development. *J Ped Gastro Nutr* 94;18:32-36

Tomblin, J.B. et al. Epidemiology of specific language impairment: prenatal and perinatal risk factors. *J Commun Disord* 1997;30(4):325-44

Victora CG et al. Evidence for protection by breastfeeding against infant deaths from infectious diseases in Brazil, The Lancet, Aug. 7, 1987: 319-322.

Williams RD, "Breast-Feeding Best Bet for Babies"

U.S. Food and Drug Administration Statement:
http://www.fda.gov/fdac/features/895_brstfeed.html

A.A.P. Breastfeeding Policy Statement: Breastfeeding and the Use of Human Milk (RE2729) Based on the research, breastfeeding for a total of 12 to 24 months can reduce your risk of ovarian cancer by about one-third.

Koletzko S, Sherman P, Corey M, et al. "Role of infant feeding practices in development of Crohn's disease in childhood." Br Med J. 1989;298:1617-1618

Young, T.K. et al. Type 2 Diabetes Mellitus in children. Arch Pediatr Adolesc Med 2002; 156(7): 651-55

Virtanen et al: "Diet, Cow's milk protein antibodies and the risk of IDDM in Finnish children." Childhood Diabetes in Finland Study Group. Diabetologia, Apr 1994, 37(4):381-7

Wiggins, PK , Dettwyler, KA" Breastfeeding: A Mother's Gift", July 1, 1998 ed., Chapter 1, L.A. Publishing Co.

Duncan, B et al "Exclusive breastfeeding for at least four months protects against Otitis Media", Pediatrics 91(1993): 897-872

Horn, RS et al "Comparison of evoked arousability in breast and formula fed infants." 2004 Arch Dis Child.; 89(1):22-25

Alm et al, "Breastfeeding and the Sudden Infant Death Syndrome in Scandanavia." June 2002 Arch of Dis in Child. 86: 400-402.

McVea, KL et al "The role of breastfeeding in sudden infant death syndrome." J Hum Lact. 2000;16:13-20

Fredrickson, DD et al., "Relationship between Sudden Infant Death Syndrome and Breastfeeding Intensity and Duration." Am. Journal of Diseases in Children, 1993: 147:460

Ford RPK, et al ."Breastfeeding and the Risk of Sudden Infant Death Syndrome." International Journal of Diseases in Children, 1993, 22(5):885-890

Taylor BJ, Mitchell EA, et al. "Breastfeeding and the risk of sudden infant death syndrome. Int J. Epidemiol. 1993;22:885-890

Scragg LK, Mitchell EA, Tonkin SL, et al. "Evaluation of the cot death prevention programme in South Auckland." NZ Med J. 1993;106:8-10

Betran et al; "Ecological Study of effect of breastfeeding on infant mortality in Latin America." Br Med J 2001; 323:1-5

Dewey KG, Heinig MJ, Nommsen-Rivers LA. "Differences in morbidity between breast-fed and formula-fed infants." Pediatr. 1995;126:696-702

Beaudry M, Dufour R, Marcoux S. "Relation Between infant feeding and infections during the first six months of life." J Pediatr. 1995; 126:191-197

Howie PW, Forsyth JS, Ogston SA, et al. "Protective effect of breast feeding against infection." Br Med J. 1990;300:11-16

Cochi SL, Fleming DW, Hightower AW, et al. "Primary invasive Haemophilus influenzae type b disease: a population-based assessment of risk factors." J Pediatr. 1986;108:997-896

Istre GR, Conner JS, Broome CV, et al. "Risk factors for primary invasive Haemophilus influenzae disease: increased risk from day care attendance and school-aged household members." J Pediatr. 1985;106:190-198

Oddy, WH et al "Breast feeding and respiratory morbidity in infancy: a birth cohort study" Archives of Disease in Childhood 2003;88:224-228

Galton Bachrach et al (2003) Breastfeeding and the Risk of Hospitalization for Respiratory Disease in Infancy" Arch Pediatr Adolesc Med 157:237-243

Grover M et al "Effect of human milk prostaglandins and lactoferrin on respiratory syncytial virus and rotavirus" Acta Paediatr. 1997; 86: 315-316

Cunningham, Allan S. MD "Breastfeeding, Bottle-feeding and Illness - An Annotated Bibliography", 1996.

Wright AL, Holberg CH, Taussig LM, et al. "Relationship of infant feeding to recurrent wheezing at age 6 years." Arch Pediatr Adolesc Med. 1995;149:758-763

Piscane A, et al "Breastfeeding and acute lower respiratory infections" Acta Paediatr. 1994; 83: 714-718

Shu X-O, et al. "Breastfeeding and the risk of childhood acute leukemia". J Natl Cancer Inst 1999; 91: 1765-72
Jacobsson LTH et al "Perinatal Characteristics and risk of rheumatoid arthritis" BMJ 2003; 326: 1068-1069

"Mother's Milk: An Ounce of Prevention?" Arthritis Today May-June 1994

"An Exploratory Study of Environmental and Medical Factors Potentially Related to Childhood Cancer." Medical & Pediatric Oncology, 1991; 19(2):115-21

Birch E, et al. "Breastfeeding and optimal visual development." J Pediatr Ophthalmol Strabismus 1993;30:33-8

Kalwart HJ and Specker BL "Bone mineral loss during lactation and recovery after weaning." Obstet. Gynecol. 1995; 86:26-32

Blaauw, R. et al. "Risk factors for development of osteoporosis in a South African population." SAMJ 1994; 84:328-32

Melton LJ, Bryant SC, Wahner HW, et al. "Influence of breastfeeding and other reproductive factors on bone mass later in life." Osteoporos Int. 1993;22:684-691

Cumming RG, Klineberg RJ. "Breastfeeding and other reproductive factors and the risk of hip fractures in elderly woman." Int J Epidemiol 1993;22:684-691

Newman, J, MD, FRCPC "How Breast milk Protects Newborns" http://www.promom.org/bf_info/sci_am.htm

Shulman et al "Early feeding, feeding tolerance and lactase activity in preterm infants." J Pediatr 1998; 133:645-649

Catassi et al "Intestinal permeability changes coloring the first month; effect of natural versus artificial feeding." J Pediatr Gastroenterol Nutr 1995; 21: 383-386

The Baby Book - Everything You Need to Know About Your Baby From Birth to Age Two c. 1992, 2003 William Sears, MD and Martha Sears, RN, Little, Brown & Co.

Armstrong, J et al, "Breastfeeding and lowering the risk of childhood obesity." Lancet 2002, 349: 2003-4

Toschke, A.M. et al, "Overweight and obesity in 6 to 14-year-old Czech children in 1991: protective effect of breast-feeding", J Pediatr Gastroenterol Nutr. 2002 Dec; 141(6):764-9

von Kries, R et al, "Breastfeeding and obesity: cross sectional study." BMJ 1999; 319:147-150 (July 17)

Rigas A, Rigas B, Blassman M, et al. "Breast-feeding and maternal smoking in the etiology of Crohn's disease and ulcerative colitis in childhood." Ann Epidemiol. 1993;3387-392

Kennedy KI, Visness CM. "Contraceptive efficacy of lactational amenorrhoea." Lancet. 1992; 339:227-230

Labbock MH, Colie C. "Puerperium and breast-feeding." Curr Opin Obstet Gynecol. 1992; 4:818-825

Riordan, J "The cost of not breastfeeding: a commentary" J Hum Lact 1997; 13(2) 93-97

A.A.P. Breastfeeding Policy Statement: Breastfeeding and the use of human milk. Pediatrics Vol. 115 No. 2 February 2005 (http://aappolicy.aappublications.org/cgi/content/full/pediatrics;115/2/496)

Acheston, L, "Family violence and breastfeeding" Arch. Fam. Med. 1995, 4:650-652

Van Den Bogaard, C. "Relationship Between Breast Feeding in Early Childhood and Morbidity in a general Population."Fan Med, 1991; 23:510-515

Owen CG et al (2002) "Infant Feeding and Blood Cholesterol: A Study in Adolescents and a Systemic Review" Pediatrics 110: 597-608 According to a study of 17,046 mother and infant pairs in Belarus, breastfed infants had a significant reduction in risk of gastro-intestinal infection

Labbok, M.H. "Does Breastfeeding Protect against Malocclusion? An Analysis of the 1981 Child Health Supplement to the National Health Interview Survey" American Journal of Preventive Medicine, 1987

Loesche WJ, "Nutrition and dental decay in infants." Am J Clin Nutr 41; 423-435, 1985

Neiva et al, J Pediatr (Rio J) 2003;79(1):07-12
Tongue thrust problems often develop among bottle-fed babies as they try to slow down the flow of milk coming from an artificial nipple. This can lead to speech problems later on.

Heacock, H.J. "Influence of Breast vs. Formula Milk in Physiologic Gastroesophageal Reflux in Healthy Newborn Infants" Jour. Pediatr Gastroenterol Nutr, 1992 January; 14(1): 41-6

Baumgartner, C.,"Psychomotor and Social Development of Breast Fed and Bottle Fed babies During their First year of Life". Acta Paediatrica Hungarica, 1984

Pisacane A, et al "Breastfeeding and Urinary Tract Infection" J Pediatr 1992 120: 87-89

Baumgartner, C., "Psychomotor and Social Development of Breast Fed and Bottle Fed babies During their First year of Life". *Acta Paediatrica Hungarica* 1984; 25(4): 409-17

4 & 5
American Academy of Pediatrics Work Group on Breastfeeding. Breastfeeding and the use of human milk. Cognitive development 1. *Pediatrics* 1997;100:1035-39.

Dunn, D. T. , M. L. Newell, A. E. Ades, and C. S. Peckham. Risk of human immunodeficiency virus type 1 transmission through breastfeeding. *Lancet* 1992; 340(8819):585-88.

Greiner, T. The HIV challenge to breastfeeding. *Breastfeeding Review* 1999; 7(3):5-9.

Hormann, E. Breastfeeding and HIV. *Breastfeeding Review* 1997; 5(2):21-24.

John, G. C. and J. Kreiss. Mother-to-child transmission of human immunodeficiency virus type 1. *Epidemiol Rev* 1996; 18(2):149-57.

Newell, M. L. , G. Gray, and Y. J. Bryson. Prevention of mother-to-child transmission of HIV-1 infection. *AIDS* 1997; 11(suppl A):S165-72.

Thiry, L. , S. Sprecher-Goldberger, T. Jonckheer et al. Isolation of AIDS virus from cell-free breast milk of three healthy virus carriers. *Lancet* 1985; 2(8583): 981.

UNAIDS/UNICEF/WHO. *HIV and infant feeding: Guidelines for decision-makers, 1998* . WHO/FRH/CHD/98.1.

UNAIDS/UNICEF/WHO. HIV and infant feeding: A review of HIV transmission through breast-feeding, 1998. WHO/FRH/NTU/CHD/98.3.

World Health Organization. Breastfeeding and replacement feeding practices in the context of mother-to-child transmission of HIV. http://www.who.int/child-adolescenthealth/publications/NUTRITION/WHO_FCH_CAH_01.21.htm

6
American Academy of Pediatrics Subcommittee on Neonatal Hyperbilirubinemia. Neonatal jaundice and kernicterus. *Pediatrics*. 2001; 108(3): 763-765.

http://www.womens-health.org.nz/breastfeed/breastlinks.htm

La Leche League International

7
Arpino C, Brescianini S, Robert E et al. Teratogenic effects of antiepileptic drugs: use of International Database on Malformations and Drug Exposure (MADRE). Epilepsia 2000 Nov;41 (11):1436-43.

Correa-Villaseanor A, Wilson PD, Loffredo C et al. Cardiovascular malformation and prenatal environmental exposures. Pediatr Res 1991 Apr;29(4 Pt 2):17A.

Correy JF, Newman NM, Collins JA et al. Use of prescription drugs in the first trimester and congenital malformations. Aust N Z J Obstet Gynaecol 1991 Nov;31(4):340-4.

Rockenbauer M, Sorensen HT et al. A population-based case-control teratologic study of ampicillin treatment during pregnancy. Am J Obstet Gynecol 2001 Jul;185(1)

Czeizel AE, Rockenbauer M. A population-based case-control teratologic study of oral oxytetracycline treatment during pregnancy. Eur J Obstet Gynecol Reprod Biol 2000 Jan;88(1):27-33.

California Birth Defect Monitoring Program. http://www.cbdmp.org/bd_heart.htm Accessed January, 2004

Centers for Disease Control and Prevention, National Center on Birth Defects and Developmental Disabilities. Autism Spectrum Disorders. www.cdc.gov/ncbddd/dd/ddautism.htm

Golding J, Vivian S, Baldwin JA. Maternal anti-nauseants and clefts of lip and palate. Hum Toxicol 1983 Jan;2(1):63-73.

Kaneko S, Kondo T. Antiepileptic agents and birth defects. CNS Drugs 1995 Jan;3(1):41-55. Kozer E, Costei A, Boskovic R et al. Association of aspirin consumption during the first trimester of pregnancy with congenital anomalies: a meta-analysis. Pediatr Res 2002 Apr;51(4 Pt 2):68A-69A.

Kricker A, Elliott JW, Forrest JM, McCredie J. Congenital limb reduction deformities and use of oral contraceptives. Am J Obstet Gynecol 1986 Nov;155(5):1072-8.

Nora AH, Nora JJ. A syndrome of multiple congenital anomalies associated with teratogenic exposure. Arch Environ Health 1975 Jan;30(1):17-21.

Saxen I. Associations between oral clefts and drugs taken during pregnancy. Int J Epidemiol 1975 Mar;4(1):37-44.

8
www.Dr.VernonColeman.com
www.cancernet.co.uk

9
Grodstein F, Goldman MB, Ryan L, Cramer DW. Relation of female infertility to consumption of caffeinated beverages. Am J Epidemiol. 1993 Jun 15;137(12):1353-60.

Wilcox A, Weinberg C, Baird D. Caffeinated beverages and decreased fertility. Lancet. 1988 Dec 24-31;2(8626-8627):1453-

Olsen J. Cigarette smoking, tea and coffee drinking, and subfecundity. Am J Epidemiol. 1991 Apr 1;133(7):734-9.

Watkins ML, Rasmussen SA, Honein MA, Botto LD, Moore CA. Maternal obesity and risk for birth defects. Pediatrics. 2003 May;111(5 Part 2):1152-8.

Castro LC, Avina RL Maternal obesity and pregnancy outcomes. Curr Opin Obstet Gynecol. 2002 Dec;14(6):601-6.

Ball TM & Wright AL. Health care costs of formula-feeding in the first year of life. *Pediatrics* 1999-4;103(4)pt2:870-76

Birch, E. et al. Breast-feeding and optimal visual development. *J Ped Ophthal Strab* 1993; 30 (1):33-38.

Horwood, L.J. et al. Breastfeeding and later cognitive and academic outcomes. *Pediatrics* 1998; 101(1):e9.

10
Report No. 086 - Biological Effects and Exposure Criteria for Radiofrequency Electromagnetic Field
Report No. 86 presents the results of a comprehensive evaluation of the available literature on the biological effects of radiofrequency electromagnetic fields. This Report begins with a discussion of studies of biological effects at the molecular level and continues to progressively larger scales of interaction, covering macromolecular and cellular effects, chromosomal and mutagenic effects and carcinogenic effects. The Report then goes on to treat systemic effects such as those relating to reproduction, growth and development, hematopoesis and immunology, endocrinology and the autonomic nerve function, cardiovascular and cerebrovascular effects, interaction of electromagnetic fields with the central nervous system and the special senses. The Report treats neurological effects and assesses studies relating to behavioral effects. The careful evaluation of the research studies forms the basis for the exposure criteria enunciated in the Report. These specify permissible levels, not only for individuals exposed occupationally, but for members of the general public exposed to radiofrequency electromagnetic radiation.

www.gsm.org/health/links/independent.shtml

11
Bottle-fed babies are at increased risk of cardiopulmonary disturbances, including prolonged airway closure and obstructed respiratory breaths due to repeated swallowing. According to one study, infants can experience oxygen saturation below 90% when bottle feeding. Nine of 50 healthy term infants in one study experienced bradycardia during bottle feeding. Six of these episodes were preceded by apnea, three showed hypopnea (marked reduction in ventilation) and one had certral apnea (no respiratory efforts).

Koenig HS, Davies Am, Thach BT. "Coordination of breathing, sucking and swallowing during bottle feedings in human infants." J Appl Physiol 69: 1629: 1623-1629, 1990.

Matthew O, Clark ML, Ponske MH. Apnea, bradycardia, and cyanosis during oral feeding in term neonates." J Pediatr 106:857, 1985

12
http://www.aap.org/breastfeeding/bppophist.cfm

13
Collaborative Group on Hormonal Factors in Breast Cancer (2002). "Breast cancer and breastfeeding: collaborative reanalysis of individual data from 47 epidemiological studies in 30 countries, including 50,302 women with breast cancer and 96,973 women without the disease." Lancet 360: 187-95

Dettwyler KA. Cutting Breast Cancer Risk: Reason to Breastfeed. *Leaven.* 1999 Apr-May;35 (2):29.
http://www.lalecheleague.org/lllleaderweb/LV/LVAprMay99p29.html

Freudenheim JL, Marshall JR, Vena JE, Movsich KB, Muti P, Laughlin R, Nemoto T, Graham S Lactation history and breast cancer risk. *Am J Epidemiol.* 1997 Dec;146(11):932-8.

Lee SY, Kim MT, Kim SW, Song MS, Yoon SJ. Effect of lifetime lactation on breast cancer risk: a Korean women's cohort study. *Int J Cancer .* 2003 Jun 20;105(3):390-3.

Zheng, T.; Duan, Li; Liu, Yi; Zhang, Bing; Wang, Yan; Chen, Yongxiang; Zhang, Yawai; and
    Owens, P.H.. (2000). Lactation Reduces Breast Cancer Risk in Shandong Province,
    China. *Am. J. Epidemiology*, 152 (12):1129-1135.

14

Barone JG, Ramasamy R, Farkas A, Lerner E, Creenan E, Salmon D, Tranchell J, Schneider D.
Breastfeeding During Infancy May Protect Against Bed-wetting During Childhood. Pediatrics.
2006. Published online June 2006, doi: 10.1542/peds.2005-2738.

15
Source: Nielsen Research Multimedia System
Source: Department of Health answer to PQ tabled by Annette Brooke MP on 26/03/07

16
Rachel's Environment and Health Weekly, No.454, August 10, 1995.

17
American Academy of Paediatrics, vol. 115, no.3, March 2003, 269-276 - Pre-term infants who
are given breast milk are protected against septicaemia.

Raisler J et al. Breast-feeding and infant illness: A dose-response relationship? *Am J Publ Hlth*
1999-1; 89(1):25-30.

Riordan J The cost of not breastfeeding: A commentary. *J Hum Lact* 1997;13(2):93-97.

18
Singhal A, Cole TJ, Lucas A. "Early nutrition in preterm infants and later blood pressure: two
cohorts after randomised trials." *Lancet* 2001 Feb 10;357(9254):413-9
Exclusive breast feeding seems to have a protective effect against some risk factors for cardiovascular disease in later life.

19
Lvoff-NM et al. Effect of the baby-friendly initiative on infant abandonment in a Russian hospital. Archives-Of-Pediatrics-And-Adolescent-Medicine. MAY 2000; 154(5):474-477.

Acheson, L., "Family Violence and Breast-feeding" Arch Fam Med July 1995; Vol 4,pp 650-652.

Lane Strathearn, MBBS, FRACP at the November 2003 AAP Section on Breastfeeding Educational
Program. Breastfeeding and Mother-Infant Separation: Independent Predictors of Child Abuse
and Neglect

20
www.who.int

21
Akre, J. (Ed.) (1992). Infant feeding the physiological basis. Geneva: World Health Organization.

Bachrach, Virginia; Schwartz, Eleanor; Bachrach, Lela (2003). Breastfeeding and the Risk of
Hospitalization for Respiratory Disease in Infancy. *Arch Pediatr Adolesc Med*, 157: 237-243

Ball TM; Wright AL (1999). Healthcare Costs of Formula-Feeding in the First Year of Life. *Pediatrics*, 103: 870-876.

Beaudry M; Dufour R; Marcoux S (1995). Relation Between Infant Feeding and Infections During the First 6 Months of Life. *Journal of Pediatrics*, 126:191 - 197.

Bener A; Denic S; Galadari S (2001). Longer Breast-Feeding and Protection Against Childhood Leukamia and Lymphomas. *Eur J Cancer* 37 (2): 234-238.

Blom L; Dahlquist G; Lonnberg G (1991). The Swedish Childhood Diabetes Study: A Multivariate Analysis of Risk Determinants for Diabetes in Different Age Groups. *Diabetologia 34*: 757-762.

Dewey K (2003). Is Breastfeeding Protective Against Childhood Obesity? *J Hum Lact.* 19 (1): 9-18.

Gerstein, Hertzel C (1994) Cow's Milk Exposure and Type I Diabetes Mellitus. A Critical Overview of the Clinical Literature. *Diabetes Care* 17:13-19.

Hardell L; Dreifaldt AC (2001). Breastfeeding Duration and the Risk of Malignant Diseases in Childhood in Sweden. *Eur J Clin Nutr* 55: 179-185.

Hoey C; Ware JL. (1997). Economic Advantages of Breast-Feeding in an HMO: Setting a Pilot Study. *Am J Manag Care*, 3: 861-865.

Howie PW; Forsyth JS; Ogsten SA; Clark A; Florey CD (1990). Protective Effect of Breast Feeding Against Infection. *BMJ*, 300: 11-16.

La Leche League International

Nafstad P; Jaakkola JJ; Hagen JA; Botten G; Kongrud J (1996). Breastfeeding, Maternal Smoking, and Lower Respiratory Tract Infections. *Eur Respir J*, 9:2623-2629.

Norris, Jill; Fraser, Scott (1995) A Meta-Analysis of Infant Diet and Insulin-Dependent Diabetes Mellitus: Do Biases Play a Role? *Epidemiology* 7 (1): 87-92.

Oddy WH; Holt PG; Sly PD, et al (1999). Association Between Breast Feeding and Asthma in 6-Year-Old Children: Findings of a Prospective Birth Cohort Study. *BMJ*, 319: 815-819.

Raisler, Jeanne; Alexander, Cheryl; O'Campo, Patricia (l999). Breast-Feeding and Infant Illness: A Dose-Response Relationship? *American Journal of Public Health*, 89 (13: 2530.

Toschke, Andre Michael; Vignerova, Jana; Lhotska, Lida; Osancova, Katerina; Koletzko, Berthold; von Kries, Rudiger (2002). Overweight and Obesity in 6- to 14-Year-Old Czech Children in 1991: Protective Effect of Breast-Feeding. *Journal of Pediatrics* 141 (6): 764-769.

UK Childhood Cancer Study (UKCCS) *BR J Cancer* Nov 30, 2001; 85(11): 1685-94.
World Health Assembly (2003). *Global strategy for Infant and young child feeding*. Geneva:World Health Organisation www.who.int

Palti et al., "Episodes of illness in breast-fed and bottle-fed infants in Jerusalem," Israel Journal of Medical Science (Israel) 20, no. 5 (May 1984): 395-9.

Victora et al., "Infant feeding and deaths due to diarrhea. A case-control study," American Journal of Epidemiology (Brazil) 129, no. 5 (May 1989): 1032-41

Howie et al., "Protective effect of breast feeding against infection," British Medical Journal (Scotland) 300, no. 6716 (Jan 6, 1990): 11-6.

Sachdev et al., "Does breastfeeding influence mortality in children hospitalized with diarrhoea?" Journal of Tropical Pediatrics (India) 37, no. 6 (Dec 1991): 275-9.

Beaudry et al., "Relation between infant feeding and infections during the first six months of life," Journal of Pediatrics (Canada) 126, no. 2 (Feb 1995): 191-7.

Lopez-Alarcon et al., "Breast-feeding lowers the frequency and duration of acute respiratory infection and diarrhea in infants under six months of age," J Nutr (Mexico) 127, no. 3 (Mar 1997): 436-43.

Victora et al., Evidence for protection by breastfeeding against deaths from infectious diseases in Brazil. Lancet (Brazil) 2, no. 8554 (Aug 1987): 319-22.

Pisacane et al., "Breastfeeding and acute lower respiratory infection," Acta Paediatr (Italy) 83, no. 7 (Jul 1994): 714-8.

Lopez-Alarcon et al., "Breast-feeding lowers the frequency and duration of acute respiratory infection and diarrhoea in infants under six months of age," J Nutr (Mexico) 127, no. 3 (Mar 1997): 436-43.

Cesar et al., "Impact of breast feeding on admission for pneumonia during post neonatal period in Brazil: nested case-control study," British Medical Journal (Brazil) 318, no. 7194 (May 1999): 1316-20.

von Kries et al., "Breast feeding and obesity: cross sectional study," British Medical Journal Germany) 319,no.7203(July17,1999)147-50.

One and a half million lives could be saved every year by reversing the decline in breast-feeding, says the United Nations Children's Fund (UNICEF): Children who are exclusively breast-fed for at least 6 months are half as likely to develop cancer before the age of 15 than children not breastfed. In southern Brazilian cities babies who receive no breast milk are 14.2 times more likely to die from diarrhoea than breastfed babies. Children who receive cow's milk formulas before the age of 2 months are twice as likely to develop diabetes.

Non-breastfed infants are almost 3 times more likely to be victims of sudden infant death than breastfed infants. Among breastfed children, the longer the duration of breastfeeding, the lower the incidence of malocclusion. From birth to 6 months bottle-fed infants are 5 times more likely than breastfed infants to contract urinary infections. Infants aged from birth to 12 months who are exclusively breastfed have one half the number of ear infections than infants who are not breastfed.

Children who have been breastfed show fewer decayed deciduous teeth than children not breastfed. Both pre-term and full-term breast milk-fed infants have better vision at 4 months and at 36 months than artificially fed infants. Children breastfed for longer periods showed higher scores on mental ability tests. Bottle-fed infants have increase rates of ARI. Multiple sclerosis victims are less likely to have been breastfed than healthy people.

22
Biering G, Karlsson S, Clark NC, Jonsdottir KE, Ludvigsson P, Steingrimsson O. Three cases of neonatal meningitis caused by Enterobacter sakazakii in powdered milk. J Clin Microbiol 1989;27:2054-6

Dabeka RW, McKenzie AD. Lead and cadmium levels in commercial infant foods and dietary intake by infants 0-1 year old. Food Additives and Contaminants 1988;5:333-42

Koo WWK, Kaplan LA, Krug-Wispe SK. Aluminum contamination of infant formulas. J Parenteral Enteral Nutrition 1988;12:170-3

Mytjens HL, Roelofs-Willemse H, Jaspar GHJ. Quality of powdered substitutes for breastmilk with regard to members of the family Enterobacteriace. J Clin Microbiol 1988;26:743-6

Westin JB. Ingestion of carcinogenic N-nitrosamines by infants and children. Arch Environmental Health 1990;45:359-63

Babbit, V, "FDA Recalls Baby Formula, 1998", Breastfeeding.com, Inc.

23
www.babymilkaction.org
"Formula Recalls," Mothering, January-February 1998, pp. 62-63.

24
Maureen Minchin, Breastfeeding Matters, 1998 edition page 20

Food Chemical News
September 20 1982; July 11 1983 page 15; September 12 1983 page 25; October 17 1983 page 7 October 24 1983 page 40

Food Chem.Toxic.
1982 20, 5, 939 - 44

Havery, D.C. T. Fazio *Estimation of volatile N - Nitrosamines in rubber nipples of baby bottles.*

25
Radford, A., "The Ecological Impact of Bottle Feeding," Breastfeeding Review (May 1992): 204-208.

26
www.rainforestfoundationuk.org

27
Touching: the human significance of skin, Ashley Montague
The Biology of Transcendence: a blueprint of the human spirit, Joseph Chilton Pearce
Breastfeeding is essential for bio-psycho-spiritual health, Pam Chubbuck, PhD
Molecules of emotion, Candace Pert
Core energetics, John Pierrakos, MD
Bioenergetics, Alexander Lowen, MD

28
Renee Spitz (1946/1965) documented that infants isolated in cribs with little or no physical contact & physical affection can die from an emotional wasting away, which he called marasmus, even though medical & physical care were normal.

Montagu (1971) has provided a history of 2 national historical sources that have opposed bonding in the mother-infant/child relationship & which established wrongful child rearing practices in America for this past century & which continues to this day.

Montagu, A. (1971). *Touching: The Human Significance of the Skin.*
  Columbia University Press

Prescott, J.W. (1968). Early Social Deprivation. Chapter IV. IN: *Perspectives on Human Deprivation: Biological, Psychological, and Sociological.*

29
Brams M and Maloney J. "Nursing bottle caries" in breastfed children. J Peds 103(3): 415-416, 1983.

Erickson PR, Mazhari E. Investigation of the role of human breast milk in caries development. *Pediatr Dent* 1999 ZMar-Apr;21(2):86-90.·

Gardner DE, Norwood JR, Eisenson JE. At-will breastfeeding and dental caries: four case ports. ASDC J Dent Child May-Jun 1977, 1-6.

Geneva Infant Feeding Action, Post Box 157, 1211 Geneva 19, Switzerland

Gupta et al., "Reversal of Fluorosis in Children." Acta Paediatr Jpn 38, Brian Palmer, "Breastfeeding and Infant Caries: No Connection," ABM News and Views 6, no. 4 (2000): 27.

Mohan et al., "The relationship between bottle usage/content, age and number of teeth with mutans streptococci colonization in 6-24-month-old children," Comm Dent Oral Epidemiol 26, no. 1 (Feb. 1998): 12-20.

Woolridge, M., and Baum, J.D. The regulation of human milk flow. Perinatal Nutrition, Vol 6, ed. BS Lindblad. London: Academic Press, 1988.

Woolridge, M. Anatomy of infant sucking. Midwifery 2: 164-171, 1986.

30
Pertez and Kafka, "Baby Bottle Tooth Decay and Complications during Pregnancy and Delivery," Pediatric Dentistry 19, no. 1 (1997): 34-36.

31
Dr. Francis M. Pottenger, Jr., *MD* http://www.ppnf.org
Dr. Weston Price was a dentist who travelled around the world in the 1930s and 1940s studying the diets of primitive people isolated from the modern world. He found that he could eliminate or greatly reduce bad bacteria in the mouth, the supposed cause of tooth decay through diet alone. Tooth decay begins many generations back.

When Dr. Price analyzed the foods used by isolated primitive people he found that they provided at least four times the water soluble vitamins, calcium and other minerals, and at least TEN times the fat soluble vitamins from animal foods such as butter, fish eggs, shellfish and organ meats... Many tribes required a period of premarital nutrition, and children were spaced to permit the mother to maintain her full health and strength, thus assuring subsequent offspring of physical excellence. Many primitive groups Dr. Price studied had a tooth cavity rate close to zero. Weston Price also noticed in groups following their traditional diet that decayed teeth either fell out painlessly, or they covered themselves over with a hardened layer of enamel.

Not eating enough nutrients isn't the only reason why teeth would decay. They also could decay because the body has become too toxic. This is highly likely with formula milk as the body does not recognise it as a 'food'.

32
Speller E 2000, Breastfeeding and Dental Caries. NMAA Hot Topic 5: 1-4.

33
New sustainable plant source of omega-3. 27 March 2007, PR49/07
http://www.kcl.ac.ukphpnews/wmview.php?ArtID=1770

34
Prescott, J.W. (1997). Breastfeeding: Brain nutrients in brain development for human love and peace. Touch the Future. Spring . http://www.violence.de/prescott/ttf/article.html
Prescott, J.W.(2002) How Culture Shapes the Developing Brain .Touch the Future . Spring http://violence.de/prescott/ttf/cultbrain.pdf

35
Allen DA. Autistic spectrum disorders: clinical presentation in preschool children. J Child Neurol. 1988;3 Suppl:S48-56.

al-Jarallah AA, Salih MA, al Nasser MN, al Zamil FA, al Gethmi J. Rett syndrome in Saudi Arabia: report of six patients Ann Trop Paediatr. 1996 Dec;16(4):347-52.

Batshaw ML, Hyman SL, Mellits ED, Thomas GH, DeMuro R, Coyle JT. Behavioral and neurotransmitter changes in the urease-infused rat: a model of congenital hyperammonemia. Pediatr Res. 1986 Dec;20(12):1310-5.

Benno Y, Mitsuoka T. Impact of Bifidobacterium longum on human fecal microflora. Microbiol Immunol. 1992;36(7):683-94.

Butel MJ, Roland N, Hibert A, Popot F, Favre A, Tessedre AC, Bensaada M, Rimbault A, Szylit O. Clostridial pathogenicity in experimental necrotising enterocolitis in gnotobiotic quails and protective role of bifidobacteria. J Med Microbiol. 1998 May;47(5):391-9.

Levy PQ, Bicho MP. [Platelet serotonin as a biological marker of autism] [Article in Portuguese] Acta Med Port. 1997 Dec;10(12):927-31

Lok E The effect of weaning on blood, hair, fecal and urinary mercury after chronic ingestion of methylmercuric chloride by infant monkeys. Toxicol Lett. 1983 Feb;15(2-3):147-52.

Morishita Y, Shiromizu K. Effects of dietary lactose and purified diet on intestinal microflora of rats. Jpn J Med Sci Biol. 1987 Feb;40(1):15-26.

Nishikawa I, Kawanishi G, Cho F, Honjo S, Hatakeyama T. Chemical composition of cynomolgus monkey milk. Jikken Dobutsu. 1976 Oct;25(4):253-64.

Picaud JC Formula-fed preterm neonates Minerva Pediatr. 2003 Jun;55(3):217-29.

Qazzaz ST, Mamattah JH, Ashcroft T, McFarlane H. The development and nature of immune deficit in primates in response to malnutrition. Br J Exp Pathol. 1981 Oct;62(5):452-60

Sandler RH, Finegold SM, Bolte ER, Buchanan CP, Maxwell AP, Vaisanen ML, Nelson MN, Wexler HM. Short-term benefit from oral vancomycin treatment of regressive-onset autism. J Child Neurol. 2000 Jul;15(7):429-35.

Sweeten TL, Posey DJ, Shankar S, McDougle CJ. High nitric oxide production in autistic disorder: a possible role for interferon-gamma. Biol Psychiatry. 2004 Feb 15;55(4):434-7

Wagner JD, Jerome CP, Adams MR. Gluten-sensitive enteropathy in a cynomolgus monkey. Lab Anim Sci. 1988 Oct;38(5):592-4.

Wako H, Hatakeyama T, Kamihara M, Wada S. [Artificial nursing of new-born cynomolgus monkeys as a model of the human infant and development of abnormal behavior (author's transl)] [Article in Japanese] Jikken Dobutsu. 1975 Oct;24(4):161-71.

36

Haider R et al. (1996). Breast-feeding counselling in a diarrhoeal disease hospital. *Bulletin of the World Health Organization,* 74:713-719.

Haider R et al. (2000). Effect of community-based peer counsellors on exclusive breastfeeding practices in Dhaka, Bangladesh: a randomized controlled trial. *Lancet,* 356:1643-1647.

Haider R et al. (2002). Training peer counsellors to promote and support exclusive breastfeeding in Bangladesh. *Journal of Human Lactation,* 18:7-12.

37
Taren D, Chen J 1993, A Positive association between extended breast-feeding and nutritional status in rural Hubei Province, Peoples Republic of China. Am J Clin Nutr 58(6): 862-867.

Prentice A 1991 Breastfeeding and the older infant. Acta Paediatr Scand Suppl 374:78-88.

Prentice A 1994, Extended breast-feeding and growth in rural China. Nutr Rev 52(4): 144-146.

38
Haggerty PA, Rutstein SO 1999, Breastfeeding and Complementary Infant Feeding, and the Postpartum Effects of Breastfeeding. DHS Comparative Studies No 30, Calverton, Maryland: Macro International Inc.

39
Fawzi WW, Herrera MG, Nestel P, el Amin A, Mohamed KA 1998, A longitudinal study of prolonged breastfeeding in relation to child undernutrition. Int J Epidemiol 27(2): 255-260.

40
Rogan WC and Gladen BC 1993, Breastfeeding and cognitive development. Early Hum Dev 31:
181-193.

41
Horwood LJ, Darlow BA, Mogridge N 2001, Breast milk feeding and cognitive ability at 7-8 years
Arch Dis Fetal Neonatal 84: F23-F27.

42
Kries R von, Koletzko B, Sauerwald T, Mutius E von 2000, Adv Exp Med Biol 478: 29-39.

43
Fisher JO, Birch LL, Smiciklas-Wright H, Picciano MF 2000 Breastfeeding through the first year
predicts maternal control in feeding and subsequent toddler energy intakes. J Am Diet Assoc
100(64): 641-646.

44
Boulton J, Landers M 1999, The Toowoomba Children's Nutrition Study 1993-1997. Darling
Downs Public Health Unit, Toowoomba.

45
World Health Organisation

46
Backstrom MC, Maki R, Kuusela A, Sievanen H, Koivisto A, Koskinnen M, Ikonen RS, Maki M
1999, The long term effect of early mineral, vitamin D, and breast milk intake on bone mineral
status in 9 to 11-year-old children born prematurely. J Pediatr Gastroentrol Nutr 29: 575-582.

47
Ainsworth MA 1973, The development of infant-mother attachment. In Caldwell BM, Ricciuti
HN (eds): Review of Child Development Research, University of Chicago Press, Chicago.

48
Fergussen DM, Woodward LJ 1999, Breast feeding and later psychosocial adjustment. Paediatr
Perinatol Epidemiol 13: 144-157.

49
Zheng T, Duan L, Liu Y, Zhang B, Wang Y, Chen Y, Zhang Y, Owens PH 2000, Prolonged lactation reduces breast cancer risk in Shandong Province, China. Am J Epidem 152: 1129-1135.

50
Margot Sunderland, Director of Centre for Child Mental Health London. The Science of Parenting – she bases her work on 800 studies which show children should be able to sleep with their
parents until they're five.

51
CR Gale, CN Martyn, Lancet 1996 20:347
Breastfeeding, dummy use and adult intelligence

52
La Leche League

53
See the work of Pam Chubbuck for further information.
Breastfeeding is essential for bio-psycho-spiritual health, Pam Chubbuck, PhD

54
Read the book *Dressed to Kill ~ the link between breast cancer and bras,* by Sydney Ross Singer and Soma Grismaijer.

55
Centers for Disease Control and Prevention, National Center on Birth Defects and Developmental Disabilities. Autism Spectrum Disorders. www.cdc.gov/ncbddd/dd/ddautism.htm

56
Prescott, J.W. (1968). Early Social Deprivation. Chapter IV. IN: *Perspectives on Human Deprivation: Biological, Psychological, and Sociological.*

57
Von Kries and Hanawa 1993

58
www.aims.org.uk
Sara Wickham

59
La Leche League
Also, anecdotal evidence from breastfeeding counsellors worldwide

60
Riordin, J. 1991

61
Breastfeeding: brain nutrients in brain development for human love and peace. See table 1, James Presccott's www.violence.de/prescott.ttf/article.html

Further references
Detwyler K 1995, A time to wean. In Stuart-Macadam P, Dettwyler K (eds) Breastfeeding Biocultural Perspectives. Aldine De Gruyter, New York.

WHO (2001). The Optimal Duration of Exclusive Breastfeeding. Results of a WHO systematic review.Note for the Press #7.Geneva, http://www.who.int/inf-pr-2001/en/note2001-07.html.

Tropical Paediatrics, 1989;4:226-232 - Showed breast milk contains 'significant' antibodies to whooping cough, HIB, strep B and meningitis.

Journal of Epidemiology, 1997, 26:443-50 - Said breast milk protects against HIB meningitis for up to 10 years after breast feeding has CEASED.

Journal of Paediatrics, 29, 1962 (by Albert Sabin, inventor of polio vaccine): 'Anti-poliomyelitic activity of human and bovine colostrum and milk' - He infected mice with polio virus and then fed them human breast milk which killed the polio virus. It also killed yellow fever, dengue fever, Japanese encephalitis and West Nile virus.

Brams M and Maloney J. "Nursing bottle caries" in breastfed children. J Peds 103(3): 415-416, 1983.

Gardner DE, Norwood JR, Eisenson JE. At-will breastfeeding and dental caries: four case ports. ASDC J Dent Child May-Jun 1977, 1-6.

A.A.al-Dashti et al., "Breast feeding, bottle feeding and dental caries in Kuwait, a country with low-fluoride levels in the water supply," Community Dent Health (England) 12, no. 1 (March 1995): 42-7

A.L. Hallonsten et al., "Dental caries and prolonged breast-feeding in 18-month-old Swedish children," Int J Paediatr Dent (Sweden) 5, no. 3 (Sep 1995): 149-55.

Iacono, G. et al. Gastroesophageal reflux and cow's milk allergy in infants: a prospective study. J Allergy Clin Immunol 1996; 97(3):822-7.

Tropical Paediatrics, 1989;4:226-232 - Showed
breast milk contains 'significant' antibodies to whooping cough, HIB, strep B and meningitis. Journal of Epidemiology, 1997, 26:443-50 - Said breast milk protects against HIB meningitis for up to 10 years after breast feeding has CEASED.

Journal of Paediatrics, 29, 1962 (by Albert Sabin, inventor of polio vaccine): 'Anti-poliomyelitic activity of human and bovine colostrum and milk' - He infected mice with polio virus and then fed them human breast milk which killed the polio virus. It also killed yellow fever, dengue fever, Japanese encephalitis and West Nile virus.

Burr, C. K., S. Taylor, D. Bartelli. Reduction of Perinatal HIV Transmission: A Guide for Providers (Newark, NJ: National Pediatric and Family HIV Resource Center, 1997).

Specter, Michael, "In AIDS-Torn Africa, Desperate Choices: UN Suggestion to Stop Breast-Feeding Leaves Mothers Confused and Alarmed," International Herald Tribune, August 20, 1998, 1, 7.

Assessment of dietary vitamin D requirements during pregnancy and lactation.
Bruce W Hollis and Carol L Wagner. American Journal of Clinical Nutrition, Vol. 79, No. 5, 717-726, May 2004.

Maternal compared with infant vitamin D supplementation.
Arch Dis Child. 1986 Dec;61(12):1159-63.

Risk factors for vitamin D deficiency in breastfed newborns and their mothers.
Nutrition. 2002 Jan;18(1):47-50.

Vitamin D and mental illness by John Jacob Cannell, MD
This article lists the scientific evidence that humans need at least 3,000 IU of vitamin D daily, and also talks about the toxicity issue.

Riordan JM. The cost of not breastfeeding: a commentary. J Hum Lact 1997; 13(2):93-
Massachusetts figures were derived from national figures using population data.

Ball TM, Wright AL. Health care costs of formula-feeding in the first year of life. Pediatrics 1999; (103)4:870-66.

Cohen R, Mrtek MB, Mrtek RG. Comparison of maternal and infant illness rates among breast-feeding and formula-feeding women in two corporations. Am J Health Promot 1995; 10(2):148-53.

Chandra, RK. Five-year follow-up of high-risk infants with family history of allergy who were exclusively breast-fed or fed partial whey hydrolysate, soy, and conventional cow's milk formulas. J Pediatr Gastroenterol Nurtr 1997 Apr; 24(4):442-6.

Wafula EM, Limbe MS et al. Effects of passive smoking and breastfeeding on childhood bronchial asthma. East Afr Med J 1999 Nov;76(11):606-9.

Cognition
D. L. Johnson et al., "Breastfeeding and Children's Intelligence," Psychol Rep 79, no. 3 (December): 1179-1185.

W. J. Rogan and B. C. Gladen, "Breastfeeding and Cognitive Development," Early Human Development 3 (January 31, 1993):181-193.

M. Morrow-Tlucak, et al. "Breastfeeding and Cognitive Development in the First Two Years of Life," Soc Sci Med 26, no. 6 (1998):635-639.

C. I. Lanting et al., "Neurological Differences between 9-year-old Children Fed Breastmilk or Formula," Lancet 344, no. 8933(November 12, 1984): 1319-1322.

Child-led weaning
Katherine A. Dettwyler, "Time to Wean: The Hominid Blueprint for the Natural Age of Weaning in Modern Human Populations," in Breastfeeding: Biocultural Perspectives, P. Stuart-Macadam and K. A. Dettwyler, eds. (Aldine de Gruyter, 1995)

Pacifiers
Ollila Paivi et al., "Prolonged Pacifier-Sucking and Use of a Nursing Bottle at Night: Possible Risk Factors for Dental Caries in Children," Acta Odontol Scand 56 (1998): 233-237.

Breast cancer
Jernstorm, H et al "Breast-feeding and the risk of breast cancer in BRCA1 and BRCA2 mutation carriers." J Natl Cancer Inst. 2004;96:1094-1098

Lee, SY et al "Effect of lifetime lactation on breast cancer risk: a Korean women's cohort study." Int J Cancer. 2003;105:390-393

Collaborative Group on Hormonal Factors in Breast Cancer (2002). "Breast cancer and breast-feeding: collaborative reanalysis of individual data from 47 epidemiological studies in 30 countries, including 50,302 women with breast cancer and 96,973 women without the disease." Lancet 360: 187-95

Zheng et al, "Lactation Reduces Breast Cancer Risk in Shandong Province, China" Am. J. Epidemiol. Dec. 2000, 152 (12): 1129

The Drinks Are On Me

Neurology

Kamimura, S., Eguchi, K., Sekiba, K. (1991). Tryptophan and its metabolite concentrations in human plasma and breast milk during the perinatal period. Acta Medica Okayama. April 45 (2):101-106.

Lanting, D.I., Fidler, V. Huisman, M., Touwen, B.C., Boersma, E.R. (1994). Neurological differences between 9-year old children fed breast-milk or formula-milk as babies. (1994). Lancet. Nov 12 344(8933):1319-22.

Montagu, A. (1971). Touching: The Human Significance of the Skin. Columbia University Press

Neuringer, M. (1993). Cerebral cortex docosahexaenoic acid is lower in formula-fed than in breast-fed infants. Nutrition Reviews. August 51(8): 238-41.

Newman, J. (1995). How Breast Milk Protects Newborns. Scientific American. December. DHEW/NIH (1994). Ad Hoc Group of Consultants to the Advisory Committee to the Director, NIH. Report of the Panel on NIH Research on Antisocial, Aggressive, and Violence-related Behaviours and Their Consequences. Office of the Director, National Institutes of Health (April). Bethesda.

Prescott, J.W. (1971). Early somatosensory deprivation as an ontogenetic process in the abnormal development of the brain and behavior. In: Medical Primatology 1970 www.violence.de/prescott/mp/article.html

Prescott, J.W. (1975) Body Pleasure and the Origins of Violence. The Futurist April. Reprinted: The Bulletin Of The Atomic Scientists (1975) November. www.violence.de/prescott.bulletin/article.html

Prescott, J.W. (1990): Affectional bonding for the prevention of violent behaviours: Neurobiological, Psychological and Religious/Spiritual Determinants. Violent Behaviour Vol.I: Assessment and Intervention. (L.J. Hertzberg, et. al., Eds). PMA Publishing NY pp. 110-42

Prescott, J.W. (1996). The Origins of Human Love and Violence. Pre- and Perinatal Psychology Journal. 10(3):143-188. Spring. www.violence.de/prescott/pppj/article.html

Prescott, J.W. (2001). Only More Mother-Infant Bonding Can Prevent Cycles of Violence. Cerebrum 3(1): 8-9 & 124, Winter 2001 _www.violence.de/prescott/reviews/cerebrum.doc

Bedwetting

Barone JG, Ramasamy R, Farkas A, Lerner E, Creenan E, Salmon D, Tranchell J, Schneider D. Breastfeeding During Infancy May Protect Against Bed-wetting During Childhood. Pediatrics. 2006. Published online June 2006, doi: 10.1542/peds.2005-2738.

Cancer

Salazar-Martinez E, et al. Reproductive factors of ovarian and endometrial cancer risk in a high fertility population in Mexico. Cancer Res 1999Aug1;59(5):3658-62.

Newcomb PA, Trentham-Dietz A. Breast feeding practices in relation to endometrial cancer risk, USA. Cancer Causes Control 2000 Aug;11(7):663-7.

Bone health

Cumming RG, Klineberg RJ. Breastfeeding and other reproductive factors and the risk of hip fractures in elderly women. Int J Epidemiol 1993; 22:684-91.

Leukaemia
Shu XO, Linet MS, et al. Breastfeeding and risk of childhood acute leukemia. J Natl Cancer Inst 1999; 91(20);1765-72.

Occlusal anomalies
Karjalainen S, Ronning O, Lapileimu H, Simell O. Association between early weaning, non-nutritive sucking habits and occlusal anomalies in 3-year-old Finnish children. Int J Paediatr Dent 1999 Sep; 9(3):169-73.

SIDS
Walker, M. A fresh look at the risks of artificial infant feeding. 1993; J Hum Lact 9(2):91-107.
Ford RPK, Taylor BJ, Mitchell EA, et al. Breastfeeding and the risk of sudden infant death syndrome. Int J Epidemiol 1993;22:885-90.

Breastfeeding support groups

<u>**United Kingdom**</u>
La Leche League
PO Box 29, West Bridgford, Nottingham, NG2 7NP

Association of Breastfeeding Mothers
PO Box 207 Bridgwater, Somerset TA6 7YT
Helpline 0870 401 7711 e-mail: info@abm.me.uk

Little Angels
(01254) 772929 for breastfeeding support in East Lancashire.
Includes one to one visits at home and a daily support group at Queen's Park Hospital postnatal wards.

The Breastfeeding Network
PO Box 11126, Paisley, PA2 8YB Support line 0870 900 8787

<u>**Australia**</u>
Association of Breastfeeding Mothers
PO Box 4000, Glen Iris, 3146 Victoria
Australia
Ph: (03) 9885 0855 e-mail:

info@breastfeeding.asn.au
Breastfeeding help lines
Victoria (03) 9885 0653
New South Wales (02) 8853 4999
Queensland (07) 3844 8977
South Australia & Northern Territory (08) 8411 0050
Western Australia (08) 9340 1200
Australian Capital Territory (02) 6258 8928
Tasmania (03) 6223 2609

La Leche League
PO Box 1270, Wellington
Telephone/Facsimile (04) 471 0690
E-mail lllnz@clear.net.nz
Website: www.lalecheleague.org.nz

For La Leche League groups in your country, please contact LLL international. www.lalecheleague.org

To find out how you can help campaign against the inappropriate advertising and promotion of infant formula, please contact Baby Milk Action.
www. babymilkaction.org

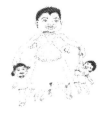

The Mother magazine

The Mother magazine was conceived when Catherine Young, the publisher and editor of my favourite parenting magazine, passed away from breast cancer. (See www.compleatmother.com ~ a magazine of natural pregnancy, birth and breastfeeding).

Her magazine had been an absolute life-line to me. I was new to England, and still a relatively young mum. Within its pages I found like-minded women and families being raised with a new consciousness. My friend, who'd been distributing The Compleat Mother, said that Catherine Young had always wanted to see a UK version of her magazine. That one sentence set off a chain of events and five months later, in February 2002, the first issue of The Mother (TM) was sent off to just 30 subscribers. That was one of the most nerve-wracking weeks of my life! However, within a week, the number of subscribers had doubled. My leap of faith had paid off. And this is how the magazine has grown ~ through passionate word of mouth. Although TM is in no way connected to The Compleat Mother, it is most certainly where the initial inspiration was drawn from, and for that I shall always be grateful.

Each issue of The Mother is gestated and birthed within the walls of our small, 300 year old, sandstone cottage at the base of the Pennines. Articles are edited, photos and illustrations chosen, and pages are laid out, all against the backdrop of our family life: the simmering of leek and potato soup in the kitchen, my girls playing with cloth dolls by the fireside, or a cat tucked up on my lap as I type; a child's fingers making music on a violin or piano; great works of art painted beside me on the dining room table, and for the first few years, breastfeeding! The essence of this grass-roots approach to a professional publication brings heart and soul to the families around the world who read The Mother.

In 2006, The Mother's family grew when The Art of Change teamed up with my family and took over the administrative and publishing arm of the magazine ~ leaving me to do what I love best, editing and design/layout.

The purpose of TM is not to prescribe a way of parenting, but to help women and men access their deep, intuitive knowing, and find a way to parent optimally. We cover many topics and aspects of natural family living ~ beginning with fertility awareness, conscious conception, peaceful pregnancy and ecstatic birthing. The natural consequences of these are: full-term breastfeeding; co-sleeping and bonded family life. We encourage natural immunity and vaccine awareness.

The Mother magazine recognises that modern technology is here to stay and aims to inform readers about how these can impact on child development.

We encourage deliberately conscious and aware consumerism, including the use of natural products (toys, cleaning and body care).

We value and recognise that children learn best in informal, child-led situations. Our articles reflect the value of small schools, forest schools and home education.

At times, most of us compromise the optimum, both in terms of parenting, and life in general. We encourage taking responsibility for the outcomes of our choices, actions and inaction.

If you've enjoyed reading The Drinks Are On Me, then I invite you to join The Mother magazine's family.

www.themothermagazine.co.uk
www.artofchange.co.uk

~ Veronika ~

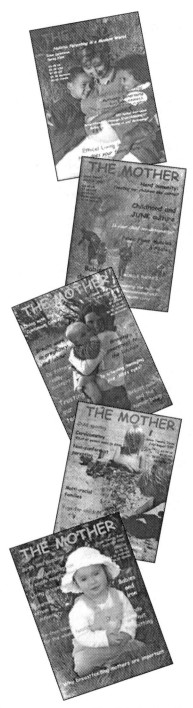

About the publisher:

The Art of Change is a publishing/production house and mail order partnership created by Barry and Winnie Durdant-Hollamby. The Art of Change seeks to help raise consciousness through the release of publications and recordings, and through the promotion of speakers and events.

In 2004 Barry and Winnie started writing for The Mother magazine – a natural parenting magazine edited by Veronika Robinson. In 2006 they were given the opportunity of taking over the publishing of the magazine, leaving Veronika to concentrate on her writing and compilation of The Mother. A year later, The Art of Change finds itself honoured to be releasing Veronika's first major book. The Drinks should really be on us!

The main objectives of The Art of Change can be summarised as:

To encourage individuals in their pursuit of happiness, and equip them with the tools to help achieve a happier and more peaceful state of being.

To help people relieve suffering and hardship caused by physical illness and emotional imbalances.

To educate individuals and organisations in the principle of taking responsibility for their own well-being.

To encourage individuals and organisations to find and achieve their own highest purposes and aspirations.

Some of the other books and recordings published by The Art of Change:

The Male Agenda
by Barry Durdant-Hollamby

The inside story on blokes. The Male Agenda challenges men who are struggling to make sense of life, to accept compromise no longer.

This book makes the prospect of change exciting and achievable, through real life stories and practical 'self-help' tools. It's also great for women wanting to understand their men.

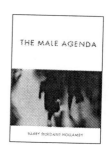

Stepping Stones

Stepping Stones is a tried and tested, easy-to-follow workbook that will help you to manage transition in your life.

Laid out in diary form, there are 84 steps to take which will walk you easily through your own unique journey. Become your own life-coach from the comfort of your recliner.

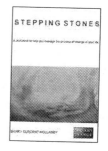

The Truth about Illness, Unhappiness and Stress?

Updated version of Barry & Winnie Durdant-Hollamby's first book on health and well-being. This revised edition contains many more case studies, and explains why our state of mind matters so much in the creation of better health.

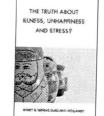

Learn to Meditate in 20 Minutes
(audio CD)

Does what it says on the box... a simple introduction for beginners. Highly recommended for anyone who's stressed.

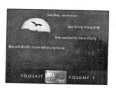

About the author:

Veronika Robinson lives in the Eden Valley, Cumbria, in northern England with her husband Paul and their two home-educated daughters, Bethany and Eliza.

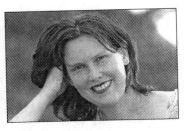

Living at the base of the Pennines, Veronika derives inspiration and nourishment from her rural lifestyle.

She founded the National Waterbirth Trust (New Zealand) in 1995, and launched The Mother magazine to an international readership in 2002. Alongside editing this unique publication on optimal parenting, Veronika's other passions include being a wife and mother, metaphysics, psychological astrology, organic gardening, living in accord with nature, self-sufficiency and music. She has worked as a spiritual celebrant since 1995.

Veronika is available for lectures and workshops, worldwide. She can be contacted via The Art of Change.

About the artist:

Andri Thwaites is passionate about horticulture and garden design. Her art includes sculptural work in gardens, pottery, ceramic and textile murals, kids' workshops, and freelance illustrative work for The Mother magazine.

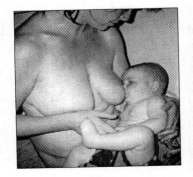

She lives with her husband Tom, and their two children, Joe Bob and Silvi, on a permaculture-inspired farm in Cumbria. She successfully breastfed both of her children.

The Drinks Are On Me

The Drinks Are On Me